Live, Work, and be Healthy

A Top Medical Director's Common-Sense Advice and Observations for the Working Person

Arthur S. Verdesca, M.D.

HEADQUARTERS MEDICAL DIRECTOR
WESTERN ELECTRIC

VNR VAN NOSTRAND REINHOLD COMPANY

NEW YORK   CINCINNATI   ATLANTA   DALLAS   SAN FRANCISCO
LONDON   TORONTO   MELBOURNE

Van Nostrand Reinhold Company Regional Offices:
New York Cincinnati Atlanta Dallas San Francisco

Van Nostrand Reinhold Company International Offices:
London   Toronto   Melbourne

Copyright © 1980 by Litton Educational Publishing, Inc.

Library of Congress Catalog Card Number: 79-19626
ISBN: 0-442-25779-1

Manufactured in the United States of America

Published by Van Nostrand Reinhold Company
135 West 50th Street, New York, N.Y.   10020

Published simultaneously in Canada by Van Nostrand Reinhold Ltd.

15 14 13 12 11 10 9 8 7 6 5 4 3 2 1

Library of Congress Cataloging in Publication Data

Verdesca, Arthur S
  Live, work, and be healthy.

  Includes index.
  1. Medicine, Popular. 2. Health. I. Title.
[DNLM: 1. Medicine—Collected Works. 2. Medicine—
Popular works. WB7 V483L]
RC81.V47   616   79-19626
ISBN 0-442-25779-1

Preface

It was in late 1965 that the first of the monthly articles that make up this book appeared in the Western Electric Headquarters employee newspaper. Those were still the days when medical topics were not big news, either in our newspapers or weekly magazines. Though the climate of publicity surrounding medical topics has changed since then, the favorable responses greeting the continued publication of these articles indicate that they still serve to fill some gaps in the layman's awareness of sickness and health, and have prompted the gathering together of most of these articles into book form.

The audience for which the articles was intended is an ambulatory, generally healthy, working population. Thus, no attempt was made to be encyclopedic. Rather, topics that would be of interest to such a population were stressed, with, for example, an omission of pediatric diseases and other topics peripheral to such a group. While the complexity and complications of medical problems that arise in a hospitalized population are sometimes alluded to in the various articles, such an emphasis was deemed, at best, tangential to the original readers of the articles. Similarly, very rare diseases are mentioned infrequently. The attempt was to cover those common conditions that can afflict the working person.

The topics are arranged under general headings, usually reflecting different body areas. The prevalence of and public interest in cardiovascular diseases account for the large number of articles in that section. The infectious disease section is large because of the great number of infections covered. However, within each of these major divisions, surely our readers will find topics omitted which they wish had been covered. We welcome their comments and suggestions.

Each brief article is so arranged as to cover a description of the disease in question, its chief presenting symptoms, and generally accepted methods of treatment. It should be emphasized that these generally accepted methods of treatment are just that—*general.* They are not intended as *specific* advice for the medical conditions that may afflict our readers. A specific problem requires specific diagnosis and specific treatment, and this is best obtained by an individual consultation with one's own physician.

Whatever faults the book has are, of course, mine. Much of the credit for whatever good things are in it is to be shared with a number of persons who were in one way or another instrumental in its publication. Thanks are therefore due to: Alexander Cohen who suggested it, and in a very special way made the whole thing possible; Emmett Nathan who guided the book's course from inception to completion; and the valiant ladies who typed it from what is rumored to be the most illegible handwriting in the world—Mae Walsh, Juneann Nakken, Catherine Davis, and Maria Rinaldi. Unique and special thanks are due to: Hilda Zambrana who organized, and copied, and reorganized, and recopied, with as much patience as all doctors should show their patients; and to my wife, Ann, who not only encouraged and tolerated, but also who read, and reread, and corrected, and clarified the manuscript. Finally a word of thanks is necessary for the gracious cooperation and encouragement received from Eugene Falken, Alberta Gordon, and Sandra Auerbach of the Van Nostrand Reinhold staff.

ARTHUR S. VERDESCA, M.D.

AN INTRODUCTION TO MY MEDICAL PHILOSOPHY

We here in America are among one of the most health conscious people in the world (probably only second to the French with their national obsession with the liver and how it affects daily health). Please note that I don't say we're one of the healthiest nations in the world; rather, one of the most health conscious. In our almost frantic pursuit of what we consider good health, we live in a state of (probably subconscious) wariness, always on the lookout for the headache, the cold, the joint pain, the diarrhea, or the constipation that "will be the death of us." The billions of dollars we Americans spend on medications to abort or to avert the above horrible, seemingly-death-dealing illnesses is truly a cause for astonishment.

Let's face it! How many people have ever really died of headaches, colds, joint aches, diarrhea, or constipation? How many people, for that matter, have every really been *seriously* incapacitated by the above-mentioned illnesses? Of course they are dis-affections, diseases of the body which cause varying degrees of temporary physical inconveniences; but since in reality they are all generally of such a minor nature, why do we react as if faced with a dreadful illness? Why do we question "the wisdom of the body?"

Perhaps the basic tenet of my medical philosophy is that the body does, indeed, have an internal wisdom in adjusting itself to conditions of health and disease that far surpasses the usually insignificant attempts at tampering with it that most of our modern medications succeed in achieving. I really believe that we Americans do not believe in our bodies. We don't trust them; we fear for them; we are afraid they won't know what to do when even minor ills upset their equilibrium. From a purely mechanistic point of view, have we ever stopped to think that in this evolutionary world of the survival of the fittest, we would long since have been wiped out as a species if our bodies were anywhere nearly as delicate and imperfect as so many of us seem to believe? If only we realize the unbelievable number and incredible complexity of the fine tuning adjustments made every minute of every hour of every day by every part of the body, then we might begin to accept with less alarm the signs and symptoms of our minor physical illnesses and distresses.

Maybe that headache is the body's *solution* to an internal set of conditions rather than the *problem* itself. Have we ever stopped to think that that cough, those sniffles, that diarrhea, those aches are *solutions* rather than *problems?* Why don't we begin to give the body the benefit of the doubt, at least for a little while?

This is not to say that the above symptoms are to be always ignored. But, how often have you had a headache that truly lasted more than 2 days? If it does, it is a most unusual headache, and rather than take some over-the-counter remedy for it, it would be much wiser to consult with a physician about such an unusual occurrence. How often does a muscular ache or pain last at a constant or increasing severity for more than a few days? If it does the latter, don't *play* doctor; *see* a doctor instead. And so with diarrhea, constipation, and the other usually minor, self-limited discomforts so many of us are subjected to every day of our lives.

Carrying this to an even more serious plane, I am emphatically for medical interferences with the wisdom of the body when it seems as if that wisdom is really breaking down. That may very well be what modern technical medicine is all about because after all we all must die; and death probably represents the ultimate overwhelming by sickness and disease of the wisdom of the body. If modern medicine can do anything to help correct *that* situation, then I feel that nothing should be spared in an attempt to restore health and prolong life.

Pneumonia is a serious infection. Sure, many people get over it by themselves; but I view pneumonia as an overwhelming of the body's forces, and I believe that medicine should be used to assist the body in righting the balance. Cancer represents a similar failure, and if we left it alone, we would die of it. If modern medicine could step in to correct that, then it should. And so on. The list of serious illnesses is almost endless, equalled only by the unlikelihood that any one of us will contract them. One day in the lives of some of us, a cancer cell may suddenly begin to grow unchecked; but that is 1 day out of thousands and thousands we will have already spent here on earth. That cancer may very well kill us; but to have lived our lives during those thousands and thousands of days in fear of what eventually did happen on one of those days is, I think, unwise. How often have you had pneumonia? How often have you had typhoid fever? How often have you had tuberculosis? How often have you had rheumatoid arthritis? And the list, indeed, is endless. What I am trying to say is that most of the time we have health, and we should act accordingly.

Contents

1
Blood

BLOOD AND BLOOD PRODUCTS

The use of blood replacement in modern medicine has become so old a procedure that many of us take it for granted and just assume that when blood is needed it's there for the asking—and in whatever quantities are required. Of course, a moment's reflection will reveal that this just is not so. There is no such thing as synthetic blood. The only manufacturer of human blood is the human body; and if so many Americans were not as generous in their blood donations as they are, the blood replacement programs would be severely hampered, not only those such as transfusions during surgery but also the "hidden" uses, many of which are literally vital for the continued good health and even lives of others.

It has only been within the past 15 years or so that the concept of fractional use of blood products has been successfully introduced into medical practice. Although prior to that whole blood was used exclusively (*whole blood* signifies blood that contains *all* of its normal components and elements), now its various components and elements can be extracted, concentrated, and used for the specific treatment of various medical conditions.

Blood plasma, the liquid portion of the blood, can usually be extracted either by letting the cells settle by gravity or through the accelerated settling caused by the rapid spinning of a centrifuge. Blood plasma itself, rather than being a simple substance, is so complex and contains so many factors that medical science has probably only begun to scratch the surface of its uses. Only those components of plasma which have been successfully extracted and are currently used will be briefly mentioned here.

The plasma is filled with many types of proteins, but the largest one is the albumin which makes up about half of the plasma content. It is successfully used, when isolated, in the treatment of certain kidney and liver ailments and also as an emergency supplement in cases of severe malnutrition. It is also often used in emergency accident cases to rapidly help treat and/or prevent shock. Plasma Protein Fraction (PPF) contains albumin plus alpha and beta globulins and is used in certain of the above conditions; and because of its higher mixture of proteins, it is more valuable than plain serum albumin.

Antihemophilic Factor (AHF) is prepared from fresh frozen plasma and has been lifesaving in helping to control the bleeding of hemophiliacs. Immune Serum Globulin (Gamma Globulin) is something with which most of us are familiar, and it has been used to modify or prevent infectious hepatitis and measles. It is also used for people who are born with a congenital lack of all gamma globulin.

Even more special among the globulins is Vaccinia Immune Globulin which has certainly saved the lives of those rare individuals who develop severe smallpox vaccination reaction. Zoster Immune Globulin is given to those people who, because of something wrong with their natural body defenses either by birth, or through sickness, or through various chemotherapies of cancer, might be developing what could very well be a life-threatening case of chickenpox. Similar immune globulins are also available for use in a comparable manner for tetanus (lock jaw), pertussis (whooping cough), and mumps.

Finally, fibrinogen is increasingly being isolated from plasma. This essential blood-clotting factor has saved the lives of many persons who were hemorrhaging because their own fibrinogen had either been destroyed or was lacking. And all this only from plasma!

Among the solid elements of whole blood (those which settle by gravity), the chief, of course, are the red blood cells. There are about 20 times as many red cells as white cells and platelets combined, and red cells can often be used as pure red cell transfusions, especially in persons whose blood volume could be dangerously overloaded if whole blood, with all its extra plasma, were to be used.

White blood cells can be separated from the other solid elements and can be used to replace those destroyed in patients by disease processes, by exposure to poisonous chemicals, and by drugs and radiation employed in the treatment of cancer and leukemia.

Finally, there are the platelets, the small but highly important solid blood elements which are critical in blood clotting and which also are used to replace any defective or missing platelets resulting from congenital or acquired diseases or secondary to treatment of various forms of cancer and leukemia.

SICKLE-CELL ANEMIA

The human red blood cell is a flat, thin, biconcave disc. It resembles, when looked at on end, a penny with central portion of both sides scooped out. The red blood cell is filled with hemoglobin which is a complex pigment molecule that can form an easily reversible bond with oxygen. The chief function of the red blood cell is to transport the oxygen (which gets into the cell's hemoglobin in the lungs) throughout the body via the arteries.

An amino acid is a relatively complex protein. It takes 574 of these various amino acids to make up one molecule of human hemoglobin. All you need is one substitution-alteration of one amino acid for another of the 574 and sickle-cell hemoglobin results. (Other substitutions result in other hemoglobin abnormalities but those are other stories.)

The sickle-cell condition presents two faces: sickle-cell trait and sickle-cell anemia. Sickle-cell *trait* occurs when only one of the two genes that determine hemoglobin structure is of the sickle variety. Sickle-cell *anemia* occurs when both genes are of the sickle variety.

Sickle-cell *trait* occurs in from 8 to 13% of black Americans. (Presently this figure is estimated to be more than 2 million people.) When their blood is tested, it will form the peculiar half-moon or sickle-shaped red blood cells that have given the condition its name. However, while it *is* true that the red blood cells in sickle-cell trait contain enough abnormal hemoglobin so that they can be made to sickle under laboratory test conditions, they do not contain enough to have sickling occur in the person. Thus, except very, very rarely, sickle-cell trait is an innocuous condition which is not associated with the anemia or other disabling conditions that are found in sickle-cell *anemia.*

Unfortunately, sickle-cell anemia is another story altogether. Luckily, it is much rarer than the trait—affecting anywhere from 0.3% to 1.5% of black Americans. It has been estimated that 45,000 to 75,000 black Americans have sickle-cell anemia, or sickle-cell disease as it is also known. These are persons who received a sickle-cell gene from both parents and who, therefore, can be considered to have a hereditary disorder.

Sickle-cell disease is such a serious condition that few persons with it live beyond age 40. It *is* true that many patients can lead reasonably normal lives, at least for long intervals. Some of them can even tolerate the persistent anemia without too many symptoms—but eventually the disease catches up with them in the form of crisis.

The sickle-cell crisis is an acute, self-limited episode of pain and fever, often without any further deterioration of the chronic anemia which is always present. No one knows for sure what precipitates a crisis, but crises seem to occur during periods when there may be some slowing of the circulation. Thus, attacks tend to occur at night or during an exposure to cold. The hallmark of the sickle crisis is the pain: in the bones, in the back, even in the large joints. This agonizing pain may remain stationary or may move from one area of the body to another. Sometimes the pain occurs in a body cavity such as the abdomen and has been mistaken for appendicitis. Generally the crisis subsides after a few days, although some patients may be left with some underlying discomfort.

Not infrequently one can detect a common body build among persons with sickle-cell *disease*. They are usually poorly developed muscularly, have a relatively short trunk with long extremities, often with unusually long, thin "spider" figures. Puberty and sexual maturation tend to be delayed, and fertility tends to be reduced. There is a definite increased susceptibility to infection, with urinary tract infections and pneumonia being especially common. For some unknown reason, osteomyelitis (a bone infection) due to an unusual bacterium, the *Salmonella,* is a unique feature of the disease.

The abnormalities of the red blood cell shape markedly decrease the efficiency of circulation of these cells. As a result, there really isn't any part of the body that is spared. Sickle-cell disease can involve the lung, the heart, the brain, the kidneys, the liver, the spleen, etc. Regardless of the variability of appearance of the above symptoms, the anemia is chronic and always present.

The outlook for sickle-cell disease is not good, with significant mortality figures occurring even in infancy. Those relatively few cases that have been surviving beyond age 40 have done so not because new treatments for the basic disease itself have been found, but because stricter attention is being paid to the prevention and treatment of infections which so often prove to be the final culprit in sickle-cell anemia.

No specific treatment is available for sickle-cell anemia. Over the years a variety of therapies have come into vogue and have then been discarded. None has yet managed to stand the test of time. Transfusions may be needed. All infections must be vigorously treated. Pain killers may have to be resorted to on a temporary basis. Patients should be cautioned against high altitudes and unpressurized planes, since the lowering of the oxygen pressure tends to foster sickling.

ANEMIA

Anemia is a condition about which much is heard in the popular media; fortunately, it is not nearly so common as the popular advertisements would have us believe. This is a good thing for people in general since, contrary to some popular opinion, anemia is not a condition to be taken lightly. In the presence of true anemia, a vigorous attempt should be made by your doctor to arrive at the correct diagnosis. The treatments of anemia are specific, different from each other, and generally do not overlap: what works in one anemia may be of no use in another. This awareness is important for in almost all cases it is necessary to actually treat the anemia rather than "let it improve with the passage of time."

In our current environment of an intelligent and medically sophisticated patient population, physicians are rarely able to fob off on kindly old Mrs. Jones a diagnosis such as "You've got a touch of anemia, my dear." Patients want to and should know quantitative degrees of anemia.

Basically, anemia is a lower than normal capacity of the blood to carry needed oxygen to the body's tissues. Since it is the hemoglobin in the blood which binds the oxygen from the lungs and carries it thoughout the body, one of the tests to determine if a person is anemic is the hemoglobin concentration of his blood. In men, a concentration of less than 14 grams of hemoglobin in every 100 milliliters of blood is considered anemia. In women, that lower limit of normal figure is 12 grams.

Since all of the hemoglobin in the blood is carried in the red blood cells, another way of determining whether or not a person is anemic is to see if his red blood cell count is lower than it should be. An adult male is considered anemic if his red blood cell count is below 4.5 million per cubic millimeter. For women that figure is 4 million.

Since there are many, many times more red cells than white cells in the blood, and since the cells in the blood are what make up the solid content of the blood, there is a third (and what many physicians consider the most reliable) anemia-detecting blood test called the hematocrit. Basically, the liquid blood is put into a centrifuge. After rapid spinning, the solid elements (which are mostly red blood cells) settle to the bottom while the plasma floats on top. The percentage of solid elements in that tube determines the hematocrit. In men, a hematocrit below 40–42% is considered abnormally low, while for women the lower limit of normal is 37%.

One obvious cause of anemia is excessive loss of blood through internal hemorrhage (such as bleeding peptic ulcer) or external hemorrhage (such as follows serious injuries). Here the case is obvious, and the treatment is equally obvious. Whole blood transfusions are needed, with blood plasma being only a temporary substitute. Surgery is sometimes needed to stop the bleeding.

Perhaps more common than these acute blood loss anemias are the chronic blood loss anemias such as can occur in a slowly oozing peptic ulcer, frequent and severe episodes of hemorrhoidal bleeding, or even unduly heavy, regular periods. Since the body can adjust more satisfactorily to a slow blood loss than a rapid one, there is usually no need for transfusions in such cases. Rather, once the case has been determined and successfully controlled, the anemia can be reversed fairly rapidly by the administration of iron, preferably by mouth. Usually by the end of 2 months, a person's blood picture is back to normal, although it is not uncommon for physicians to suggest that patients continue taking the iron medication for a total of 3 to 4 months. However, once that period is over, not only is there no need to continue taking iron regularly, but it may actually be dangerous since such excess iron is stored in the body and can cause severe damage in iron storage organs such as the liver.

Another major classification of the causes of anemia, second only to the blood loss causes listed above, are those anemias due to an actual deficiency in the bone marrow's production of red blood cells. This inadequate production can be due either to lack of necessary chemical factors that go to make up the red blood cells or to an actual failure of the bone marrow to make the cells even though all the necessary factors are present.

Iron deficiency is certainly the most common cause of anemia. It is not always due, however, to acute or chronic blood loss. During periods of rapid growth, the body needs a greater-than-usual intake of iron, and if the dietary content of iron is only marginal, anemia can result. Instances of such anemias occur in young children (especially babies who are "only milk drinkers"), young adolescent girls at the time of onset of menstruation, and in older females during pregnancy. Other cases of iron deficiency anemias can occur because the body can't absorb the normal iron content of the diet. This occurs especially in people who have had parts or all of their stomachs removed for ulcers or other reasons, as well as in persons with disorders of the small intestine. These anemias do not represent cases of chronic blood loss, but, rather, are due to inefficiency of iron absorption. Of course, the treatment for all iron deficiency anemias is the administration of iron as reviewed above, with emphasis being placed on the fact that treatment should persist only until the condition is fully corrected. No one should ever take iron regularly, indefinitely.

Our brief survey of the anemias due to deficiency of blood-forming factors concludes by mentioning two very rare deficiencies and one not so rare. The very rare ones are due to a deficiency of either copper or cobalt. Those few rare cases that have been described have occurred only in infants and have responded to supplementary doses of the missing metallic element.

The not so rare, missing-building-block type of anemia is that due to deficiency of Vitamin B-12 and/or folic acid. Since it is only practical to give Vitamin B-12 by injection, it has become one of the most abused therapies in all of medicine. The patient has to return to the doctor for treatment; the patient has to get an injection; and it bespeaks some mysterious malady which the patient is uniquely privileged to have. It is probably safe to say that the overwhelming majority of Vitamin B-12 injections given in the United States today are given needlessly. Vitamin B-12 does not help tired people; Vitamin B-12 does not help exhausted people; it does not help the nervous; it does not help the run-down. The only people it really helps are those who suffer from a Vitamin B-12 deficiency, another name for which is pernicious anemia. If you don't have true pernicious anemia, you don't need Vitamin B-12.

There are some very rare causes of Vitamin B-12 deficiency which are not due to pernicious anemia, such as infection with the fish tapeworm, certain severe chronic advanced forms of pancreatic diseases, or very, very strict fanatic vegetarianism. Since these are all relatively rare conditions, we'll concentrate on the Vitamin B-12 used for pernicious anemia. The important thing to remember is that it is a lifelong therapy. Anybody who was helped by shots of Vitamin B-12 for some months and then did not need it any longer, probably did not need it in the first place, because you need to take the shots for the rest of your life. If you don't, you may die from the disease. For so serious a disease as pernicious anemia, the requirement is one Vitamin B-12 injection per month. Those people who are getting three shots per week or per month or more often might just as well have had it squirted over the tops of their head for all the good it does them or for all the need of it they really have.

Folic acid deficiency is not uncommon. Though it resembles pernicious anemia, it is not the same thing, and the treatment is folic acid and not Vitamin B-12. Where pernicious anemia usually results from an inability of the body to absorb Vitamin B-12 because of insufficient stomach acid, the clinically similar folic acid deficiency often is due to insufficient intake of folic acid rather than to pure malabsorption. Since folic acid is found in such food items as green leafy vegetables, liver, mushrooms, etc., one has to have a fairly restricted diet to avoid coming into contact with folic acid. Interestingly enough, Vitamin C is needed in the metabolism in folic acid, so people who have severe Vitamin C disease may secondarily develop folic acid anemias. This is especially true in infants. Another common cause of folic acid deficiency is chronic alcoholism.

Among the rare vitamin deficiency anemias are pyridoxine anemia (Vitamin B-6), riboflavin (Vitamin B-2) deficiency, and pantothenic acid deficiency. These are all very rare.

Some persons develop anemia not because of a deficiency, but because of an inability of the bone marrow to make the red blood cells.

This could be caused by exposure to toxic chemicals, could be due to the unwanted side effects of anticancer chemotherapeutic agents, and could also be due to excessive exposure to radiation. There is even a congenital form of these aplastic anemias. The treatment for these anemias is very difficult, relying essentially on blood transfusions to keep the patient alive until the bone marrow resumes its blood forming function.

There is a final category of anemias in which the disorder is an excessive destruction of red blood cells. These hemolytic anemias are not at all uncommon. Some are due to hereditary enzyme deficiencies of red blood cell metabolism; others are due to abnormal shapes of the red blood cell itself. These, of course, are congenital and include such disorders as sickle-cell anemia, thalassemia, hereditary spherocytosis, and other relatively rare conditions.

A final mysterious category of anemias includes those associated with chronic diseases such as cancer, severe kidney disease, liver disease, or hypothyroidism. Here the basic problem is not the anemia itself, but the associated chronic systemic disease, and therapy, of course, should be primarily aimed at that cause.

2
Cancer

CANCER EPIDEMIOLOGY

In the past few years, much publicity was given to the Presidential campaign for an all-out attack on cancer. Some criticism of that program has been voiced in that it was analagous to carefully aiming a rifle and expecting to shoot with one "perfect shot" some deer, some birds, and some rabbits. Cancer is not just one disease, and to expect what will work for one form of cancer to be effective for others is unrealistic.

A tumor is an abnormal growth in the body. It can either be benign (the majority of them) or malignant. The latter are what we commonly call cancers. Cancer can occur in various stages. The first stage is the localized stage where the growth is limited solely to the part of the body where it arose, for example, skin, stomach, etc. The second stage would be the stage of spread to those lymph nodes which drain the involved area, to those in the neck, for example, in cancers of the mouth, and tongue, and throat, and along the lymph nodes in the breast bone and armpit in cancers of the breast. This second stage is, of course, more serious than the first stage in that it means that the cancer is beginning to spread even though the original local area may not be very massive at all. Cancers which have entered this second stage, therefore, necessarily have a lower cure rate than those which are successfully treated while in the localized stage. The third stage and the most serious is the stage of distant metastases or spreads to other organs, for example, lung cancer spreading to the bones or the brain, internal leukemia and lymphoma spreading to the skin, and so on. Cure rates in the third stage are indeed very low.

While it is true that some cancers have very serious effects because of their growth to such a size that they obstruct the vital functions of an organ, nonetheless those cancers that cause major complications to patients are those that spread widely throughout the body, usually via the lymph nodes and the blood stream. All cancers, with one exception, have this tendency to spread distantly. The exception is basal-cell carcinoma of the skin, which, though it may become very large and erode and undermine and destroy the nearby skin structures, never really spreads distantly.

The most common of all cancers is skin cancer, and fortunately it has the highest cure rate of all cancers. The manifestations of the disease are immediately evident to the patient and his doctor, resulting in rapid and often totally curative treatment. Besides the basal-cell carcinoma we have just mentioned which doesn't spread widely, there is squamous-cell carcinoma of the skin which can spread distantly and, therefore, is potentially very dangerous. Often such a cancer arises from a part of the skin which has had excessive exposure to the sun's rays and is often preceded by a special type of skin thickening called actinic or solar keratosis. The medical thrust in these cases should be less toward "trying to lock the barn door after the horse has been stolen" than toward prevention. Such prevention would consist of warning people, especially fair-skinned persons, to avoid excess sun and to have any new growth on the skin checked by a physician, even though the majority of new skin growths may be one of an almost myriad number of benign conditions.

A rare form of skin cancer, and one often dangerously malignant in that it can often spread widely while remaining quite small locally, is malignant melanoma. Some physicians believe that these melanoma moles are present from birth in afflicted persons and then become triggered for unknown reasons to grow and spread. Since this does not have a major relationship to sun exposure, the curative thrust would medically be toward early detection and treatment.

Besides implicating the sun as an environmental cause of skin cancer, recent publicity has been given to other environmental causes, such as vinyl chloride, which has been used as a propellant in commercial products. This has been shown to be probably responsible for an extremely rare form of liver cancer. Asbestos exposure is another environmental carcinogen. Rare cancers of the linings of the lungs and sometimes even the lining of the abdomen have followed significant exposure to it. Even cancer of the lung has occasionally been blamed on asbestos exposure. Of course, as we all know, cancer of the lung is indeed caused by an environmental factor in the great majority of persons—that factor being cigarette smoke. People who smoke more than one pack of cigarettes a day should be warned that they are risking cancer of the lung.

There are other forms of cancer, however, which almost seem to be hereditary. Recent publicity was given to the finding of high prevalences of stomach cancer in Minnesota, northern Michigan, Wisconsin, and the Dakotas. A closer look, however, revealed that much of the population in that area is of Scandinavian origin, and cancer of the stomach is fairly well accepted as being more common in Scandinavians than others. A hint as to why this is so is that Scandinavians tend to be largely of blood group Type A, and this has long been known to be associated with a higher frequency of pernicious anemia and cancer of the stomach; even that is not the final common pathway, though. What it is about blood group Type A that relates to cancers of the stomach is not known for sure. Is it because blood group Type A is associated with diminished production of stomach acid? It is generally medically accepted that cancer of the stomach usually is preceded by months or years, in most cases, of complete absence of stomach acid. Is it because something in the food group A people take in, combined with an associated lack of stomach acid, triggers the problem? Again, no one knows, but we are obviously far afield from trying to apply an approach that is good for cancer of the skin to cancer of the stomach.

Another group of cancers is that which is suspected of being either viral in origin or virus-assisted. Perhaps the most intensive detective work in this area is being done regarding the leukemias, the Hodgkin's diseases, and other disorders of the blood and blood-forming organs. While far from proven, there really does seem to be some evidence that viruses are potentially causative of some of these cancers.

So, we have environmental factors, internal factors, perhaps hereditary factors, and even infectious factors—all active and causative in cancer. It is a many-dimensional problem, and it is doubtful if one answer will ever be effective for all of them.

CANCER'S SEVEN SIGNALS

Cancer is one of the "big three." This year nearly 600,000 Americans will discover that they have cancer. It is second only to diseases of the heart and blood vessels as a cause of death among Americans. As a matter of fact, in children between the ages of 2 and 14 years of age, cancer is second only to accidents as a major cause of deaths. In adult females cancers of the breast, colon and uterus are the leading fatal cancers; among men they are cancers of the lung, stomach, and prostate gland.

Yet, there *is* cause for optimism. In the early 1900's few cancer patients had any hope of cure. In the late 1930's fewer than one-in-five patients was being "cured" (that is, alive 5 years after first being treated). Ten years later one-in-four cancer patients was being saved. Today the ratio is one-in-three which currently amounts to the saving of some 50,000 lives each year.

That's the optimistic side of the coin, however. The reverse side indicates that, of every four patients currently dying of cancer, one might have been saved had proper treatment been received in time. This means that of the total of 600,000 Americans who develop cancers this year, 100,000 more could be saved by early diagnosis and treatment—above and beyond the 200,000 presently cured. Another set of gloomy statistics is that cancer is the *leading* cause of death among women aged 30 to 54 and that more school children will die of cancer (about 50% due to leukemia) *than from any other disease.*

What can be done about it all?

1. Watch for cancer's warning signals.
2. Have regular checkups.

The seven classical "warning signals" are:

1. Unusual bleeding or discharge.
2. A lump or thickening in the breast or elsewhere.
3. A sore that does not heal.
4. Change in bowel or bladder habits.
5. Hoarseness or cough.
6. Unusual indigestion or difficulty in swallowing.
7. Change in size or color of a mole.

If any of these warning signals appear and persist for more than 2 weeks, a consultation with your doctor is in order. More often than not, it will not be a malignant growth, or it may be a simple precancerous condition than can be effectively treated.

The second thing we can all do about cancer is to have regular (usually annual) checkups. Abnormalities that do not appear in the above seven can often be detected by a physician either during a careful review of the patient's history, during a thorough physical exam, or as a result of special procedures or laboratory tests.

Cancers of six sites—breast, colon, lung, oral cavity, skin, and uterus—offer the greatest opportunity for saving lives, either by prevention or through early diagnosis and treatment. They add up to about 60% of all cancer cases and about 48% of deaths. The American Cancer Society has engaged in an intensive education program to save thousands of lives by concentrating especially on these areas. Their recommendations are:

1. Breast: Monthly self-examination as a regular female practice.
2. Colon and Rectum: Proctoscopic examination as routine in cancer checkups for those over 40.
3. Lung: Reduction and ultimate elimination of cigarette smoking; abstention by nonsmokers.
4. Oral: Wider practice of early detection measures.
5. Skin: Avoidance of excessive sun.
6. Uterus: Pap tests for women over 21.

Do the figures indicate that the current publicity regarding cancer is having any effect? Since 1936, the cancer death rate has fallen slowly but steadily in women, a drop of 13%. During that same interval, however, the cancer death rate has increased in men by about 37%. The most encouraging story is that for cancer of the cervix of the uterus. The number of deaths from this form of cancer has declined about 50% in one generation. The number of detected cases of this cancer has risen thanks to the wider use of the Pap test which uncovers cervical cancer earlier, before it has begun to spread. Most of these have been early cases and thus completely curable. Thus, we're seeing more such cancers (by better means of detection) and curing more.

Cancer of the lung is the most discouraging. In men it has increased more than 15 times in the past 35 years, and it is also going up in women. In between these two extremes are cancer of the breast (mortality unchanged for many years), cancer of the colon (continued improvement), cancer of the rectum (slight improvement), cancer of the larynx (continued improvement), and cancers of the prostate, bladder, lip-tongue-mouth, kidney, thyroid, and brain (plateau for last 10 years or so).

CANCER IN WOMEN

Recent surveys have shown that women with cancer have experienced more favorable survival rates than men for all the major cancer sites that occur in both sexes—as well as an improvement in the survival rates from those cancers that are found exclusively in women.

The most frequent of all cancers in women is cancer of the breast (34,500 deaths in 1978). Luckily the 5-year survival rate (which is the yardstick used by most doctors in determining cancer cures) for cancer of the breast is quite high: over 50% for all women with cancer of the breast regardless of how far it has spread at the time of initial discovery. The figures are even better—83% 5-year survival for those women whose breast cancer was localized with no evidence of spread outside the involved breast at the time of initial treatment. Much of the credit for this goes not only to the newer techniques of surgery and radiation developed in the past few decades, but also to the greater awareness of breast cancer on the part of women, to their going at, at least, yearly intervals to their doctors for checkups, and also to the recently publicized techniques of self-examination of the breast which more and more women are doing in the privacy of their homes.

However, breast cancer is indeed a formidable problem. It is the leading killer of women in the 40–44 age group, and the primary cause of cancer deaths among women of all ages. It has been estimated that one out of every fifteen women will develop this condition at some time in her life. While no female should become complacent about it, there are some who should be especially assiduous in their own monthly self-examinations and also in their physician checkups because current medical evidence would indicate that some women are more susceptible to the condition than others.

Among the factors that increase susceptibility to breast cancer are:

1. Being in the mid-40's to late-40's.
2. Being a woman whose periods began at an earlier age than average (12.8 years) and whose periods continue beyond the onset of menopause (late 40's).
3. Never having had children or not having had them until after 30 years of age.
4. Being obese.
5. Having a mother or sister who had the disease. A woman whose mother or sister has had breast cancer is twice as likely to develop the disease as a woman with no such family history. If both her mother and sister have had breast cancer, her risk may be up to 47 times greater.

Another factor that has been implicated but for which the situation is still very unclear are viruses. The normal hormones of the menstrual cycle and pregnancy have also been suspect. Even diet, which is the current American bugaboo, has been considered by some to be a factor in breast cancer causation. At one time, breast injuries were felt to be a predisposing factor to the conditon, although at present, this is no longer believed to be so. Of course, the pill has been blamed and then cleared in relation to the problem.

The ideal way a breast cancer is diagnosed is by the accidental discovery of a lump during the monthly self-examination. In essence, this is a lump that has not called attention to itself, but was rather something being looked for. It is better to examine after the period because there are, during menses, congestive lumps that appear and just as rapidly disappear once the first or second day of menses is past.

All breast lumps are not malignant. As a matter of fact, the majority of them may turn out to be a benign condition called cystic mastitis. Your doctor often can determine which is which by the history and examination you present to him. Some physicians use needle aspiration to help in the diagnosis of this breast condition.

Among the other diagnostic techniques which are widely being applied for breast cancer screening are mammography and thermography. By special X-ray techniques, mammography may be able to reveal the presence of abnormal breast tissue even before it can be felt. Thermography, a newer technique, is based on the realization that abnormally growing tissue, such as a tumor, grows at an abnormal metabolic rate, and therefore, is "hotter" than normal tissues. Thermography is, in essence, a temperature photograph of the examined area and has become a very helpful technique in diagnosis.

Currently the area of treatment of breast cancer has become very controversial. Some doctors advocate "lumpectomies" (the removal of the cancerous lump). This is probably the most controversial of the procedures in that most of the breast is left intact. Others remove the entire breast but not too much of the adjacent tissues. Finally, we have what used to be a relatively standard procedure, the radical mastectomy, which removed the entire breast, the adjoining lymph nodes, and often even associated muscle tissue. Some recent statistical studies, however, have called into question whether the long-term survival of patients is significantly improved by such a radical procedure which, of course, is usually more psychologically and physically scarring than the two less radical procedures described above. The addition of X-ray treatments to the therapy of the condition is often recommended by many physicians. Others feel that the addition of the powerful chemotherapeutic drugs will further help in checking the cancerous condition.

Perhaps the best thing that has come out of the recent publicity given to the problem is that breast cancer is no longer a taboo subject. Women are willing to speak openly about it, not only in their request for information and examination, but also in sharing with others their experiences with the disease. Groups of women, who are available to advise and reassure newly diagnosed patients, are doing much psychological good for patients who first learn of a disease that sometimes proves to be more mutilating psychologically than physically. The multipronged approach seems thus to be most effective: self-examination, consultation with your physician, and learning about the condition and its consequences from women who have also been affected.

Cancer of the uterus (with 10,700 deaths in 1978) is the second most common cancer of women. Fifty-nine percent of women with all stages, advanced or otherwise, of cancer of the uterus had a 5-year survival, while 78% experienced a 5-year survival if they had localized disease at the time of diagnosis. Some of the reasons for these good figures are that most cancers of the uterus occur in the cervix or neck of the uterus. Cells are, of course, more easily obtainable from this area than from deeper uterine areas for the so-called "Pap Smear Test" which is an examination of cells by a pathologist to see if there are any malignant or premalignant changes in them. Through this technique a greater than ever number of localized uterine cancers have been discovered and cured. More widespread use of such cervical pap smears might result in even further improvement in survival rates, which should serve as a reminder to all women—especially those over 30—to have an at-least-yearly Pap Smear.

Cancer of the stomach is number three on the list and this is a bad one indeed. Luckily (for women) it is only about half as common in women as it is in men, and luckily for everyone its actual incidence has been decreasing over the years. The reason for this actual decrease in the number of stomach cancers is unknown; at present it doesn't seem to be due to anything anybody can take any credit for. But, in spite of the decrease in incidence, the survival rates are dismally low, and a high proportion of these stomach cancers are considered inoperable. The overall survival rate is 14%, with 43% for those in whom the stomach cancer was localized.

Next on the list is cancer of the colon which occurs more often in women than men. Here the survival figures are better in women than in men, being 47% for all stages of colon cancer and 74% where the disease was localized. Much of the credit for these relatively good figures goes not only to the more radical surgery of the past two decades but also to the practice of including proctoscopic examinations as part of the yearly checkup all of those over 40 years of age should be having.

We come to the controversial lung cancer. Though, at present, it occurs five times more often in men than in women, the incidence of this dread disease is rising rapidly among women. The survival rate for all lung cancers in women is only 11% at the end of 5 years. For localized lung cancers, this figure is 40%, but, unfortunately, only one-fifth of all lung cancers in women are diagnosed at the still-localized stage. Is there anyone left in America today who hasn't heard the message that smoking is far and way the most common cause of lung cancer?

3
Cardiovascular

BLOOD PRESSURE

One thing just about everyone is interested in is his blood pressure. There seems to be something hallowed about a number, and at times people attach more significance to absolute blood pressure readings than even their doctors do. Many a person will feel better (for no good medical reason whatsoever) because his blood pressure has dropped from 136 to 134; or you'll see people looking concerned because their blood pressure differs from that magic number—90 plus your age.

Perhaps the most frequently asked question about blood pressure is: What is normal blood pressure? Unfortunately, the answer is not absolutely clear cut, and sometimes it seems to depend on which doctor you talk to. We know one thing that it isn't: It isn't 90 or 100 (or any other arbitrary number) plus your age. While certain limits are accepted by all physicians as being abnormally high, there is some real question as to when it is too low. So much has this concept of "low blood pressure" as a diagnosis of disease been questioned that most doctors nowadays believe that, short of reading so low that the patient is in shock, there is no such condition as "low blood pressure." As a matter of fact, many a physician feels that, so long as you are not in shock, the lower the blood pressure, the better.

The question remains, however: What is normal blood pressure? We can begin with a roundabout answer: Most persons who are considered to have normal blood pressure have a systolic blood pressure of 120 millimeters of mercury and a diastolic blood pressure of 80 millimeters of mercury or, in short, 120 over 80 (120/80). Agreed that lower than that figure may actually be desirable, where does one draw the line of abnormality when the figure is higher? Well, all doctors would say 240/140 is abnormal, and most doctors would say 190/110 is also too high. What about 150/90? Here one runs into real confusion: Some call this highish but normal; some would say "low abnormal." After a lot of discussion in the medical literature based on many studies on large populations, the currently accepted upper limit of normal blood pressure is 160/95. That differs from the number I was taught when I was in medical school, and it may differ from the number your own doctor was taught when he was in medical school, but it behooves us in the medical fraternity to keep up with current developments—which, in this case, are that blood pressures over 160/95 are abnormal and that some therapeutic intervention on the part of the doctor is required in all such cases.

Another question often asked is: What do these numbers actually mean? One admittedly rough approximation as to their significance would go like this: The upper number tells us about the actual pressure at which the heart is pumping blood; the lower number tells us about the condition of the blood vessels themselves. Thus, we know that the heart is pumping blood through the body at a certain pressure (usually measured in millimeters of mercury). What the doctor does when he measures your blood pressure is put a cuff on your arm and raise the pressure in it so that it exceeds the pressure at which your heart is pumping blood throughout the body. Then he listens through the stethoscope which he has previously applied over one of the large arteries on the inner aspect of the elbow. If he has, indeed, raised the pressure in the cuff to a point where it exceeds the heart's pumping pressure, then he will hear nothing; that is, he will not hear the flow of any blood through the artery. As he gradually lowers the pressure in the arm cuff, he will eventually reach a point at which it is just equal to that at which the heart is pumping blood. As he then goes slightly below that point, blood will begin to flow in a trickle through the previously closed-off blood vessel, and he will hear that flow. When he first hears the flow, he notes the pressure on the gauge. That is the systolic pressure and it tells one about the heart's pumping pressure.

The diastolic pressure is more difficult to define accurately. Imagine a pipe which is accustomed to a full flow of liquid. When it is full, one would not hear the fluid "sloshing around," but up until the time it *was* full, one would hear the sounds of turbulence. So, having heard the first (systolic) sound, the doctor keeps listening over your arm until all sounds disappear. Then, the blood vessel (the pipe) is fully relaxed and open with full flow. At this point he takes the second number—the diastolic pressure.

As many of you are doubtless aware from the publicity being given to high blood pressure (or hypertension, as it is known medically), it is a condition which can afflict as many as 15% of the adults in the U.S.A.—with women being affected twice as often as men. This figure applies to the population at large and includes sick as well as healthy persons. In an industrial situation where most of the employees are currently enjoying good health, it is, nonetheless, estimated that 6 to 10% of them may have high blood pressure, and as many as half of that 6 to 10% do not even *know* that they have hypertension.

Since the evidence indicates that hypertension is a condition that definitely should be regulated and treated if one is to avoid the very serious complications that can follow in its wake, and since the treatment of the condition is (in most cases) neither medically elaborate nor dangerous and thus is one that is within easy reach of all physicians, it is almost tragic that so many persons don't even know they have it.

The seriousness of untreated hypertension can quickly be realized when one considers the figures that indicate that cardiovascular disease is the leading cause of death in the United States today. In turn, cardiovascular disease can be broken down into two large categories: coronary heart disease and strokes. Of all the underlying causes of coronaries—and they include hypertension, abnormal levels of blood fats, diabetes, smoking, and positive family history of coronaries among others—hypertension is the most significant. To put it another way: The thing you want to avoid most of all in that list of factors is high blood pressure (and it follows that if you have some blood pressure or other abnormalities from that list, you'd be wise to concentrate, above all, in trying to bring the blood pressure under control). When it comes to the other killer of cardiovascular diseases—strokes—hypertension is so far ahead of any other causes that many physicians consider it (aside from some very rare inborn weaknesses of the blood vessels themselves) the *only* significant cause of strokes.

The causes of hypertension are many and often interrelated: underlying kidney disease, constitutional or hereditary factors, correctable abnormalities in structure of blood vessels, excess of certain body hormones, etc. Probably unusual psychological tension or one's reaction to it is also a factor, but this is much more difficult to quantitate than some of the above-mentioned factors.

What can be done about hypertension? Much. Too much, as a matter of fact, to go into detail here. Suffice it to say that by using varying doses of combinations of medicines, your doctor can lower your blood pressure down to whatever level he thinks is best—if he thinks that blood pressure should be lowered at all. While it *is* true that most blood pressures should be in the normal range, not *all* blood pressures above normal limits warrant the immediate institution of blood-pressure-lowering medications. That is a complex decision that only your doctor should make.

Finally then, one thing everyone will agree about is, "Don't *worry* about your blood pressure readings because worry and nervousness may very well raise them."

CHOLESTEROL

It's only been in the past 20–25 years that the medical profession has realized the importance of blood cholesterol as one of the predictive, causative factors in coronary heart disease. Like a high blood sugar (thus indicating diabetes or a tendency to it) and like high blood pressure, a high cholesterol has proven to be a "bad thing to have" because it's one of the most significant factors in accelerating arteriosclerosis (hardening of the arteries), which, in turn, is the factor behind most "coronaries."

For a while, in the late 1950's and early 1960's, some doubts were raised as to whether a high blood cholesterol was the bad factor or whether it was some other fatty component of the blood. That controversy has, since then, been settled pretty much to everyone's satisfaction. Yes, at least one more blood fat, the triglycerides, was implicated besides cholesterol; but cholesterol did not get off scot-free. *Both* fats are good things not to have high levels of in your blood.

Now comes the doctor's dilemma. Measuring blood cholesterol is relatively easy; measuring the other fat (the triglycerides) is quite complex. Generally, however, when one is elevated, so is the other. So doctors measure your cholesterol as an "index" of the fat status of your body.

Granted that a high blood fat content is bad (since, by definition, having a coronary is "bad"), what do you do about it to control it? More is known about cholesterol control than triglyceride control. Even though the latter is a blood fat, it seems to be related to the intake of relatively refined dietary sugars. Now, not all carbohydrates are simple sugars; starches are carbohydrates too, but they are complex carbohydrates and seem to be "okay" as far as blood fats go. (Of course, eating too many starches may make your body fat even though you don't have abnormal blood fats, but that's another problem altogether.) For those with high triglycerides, avoidance of candies, sweets, pies, soft drink beverages, and other simple sugars is usually significant in controlling *that* blood fat.

But what of blood cholesterol? This blood fat *is* influenced by the fat in your diet—specifically by the *type* of fat in your diet. Thus, corn oil, safflower oil, and even olive oil do not raise your cholesterol (although eating too much of these fats, like eating too much of anything, can make your body fat even though your blood fats are normal; and, conversely, it is *not* true that all thin people have low blood fats). Corn oil and safflower oil are the polyunsaturated type of fats you hear so much about. The "bad" fats are the saturated fats such as animal fats, including all meat fats as well as dairy fats, for, in the long run, dairy products are a form of meat product. Foods themselves high in cholesterol such as egg yolks should be limited in cholesterol-control attempts.

The body does make its own cholesterol, but eating the "right" fats can "trick" the metabolism into keeping the cholesterol under control. For specifics you should consult your own doctor, but here are some of the classical food ideas in following a cholesterol-control diet:

Avoid all visible meat fats and well fat-marbled cuts of meat—especially bad are bacon, sausages, spareribs, frankfurters, cold cuts, and average hamburger.

When eating poultry—which is generally a good thing to have— avoid poultry skin, duck, and goose.

Most fish is good, including shellfish. To be used sparingly are such fishes as salmon, herring, mackerel, trout, and sardines.

In the dairy area, not more than two whole eggs a week should be eaten, and all cream, whole milk, and whole milk cheeses should be avoided.

In the area of fats, butter, meat drippings, suet, lard, and ordinary saturated fat margarines should be avoided.

Most commercial baked goods such as cakes and pies are to be avoided unless one knows they were prepared with the right kind of fat.

Cream soups should be avoided.

All chocolates, fudge, ice cream, milk shakes, and fancy desserts should be avoided.

That list may seem discouragingly long, but if I were to list all the things you *could* eat on a cholesterol-controlling diet, the list would run on for pages.

A new cholesterol entity is High-Density Lipoprotein (HDL). At first, I was skeptical of the publicity and excitement generated by the announcement that HDL might be *the* significant factor in those cases in which elevated blood fats were significantly operative in causing cardiovascular disease. However, a review of some of the current medical literature does seem to indicate that there may be a real fire behind all that smoke. As such, it may be worth reviewing just what the HDL story is all about.

In all persons, blood fats are transported throughout the system by certain chemical protein carriers. These carriers can be distinguished among themselves by their separability according to speed of migration when subject to certain sophisticated chemical tests. The HDL spread faster across a special filter paper, followed by the low density lipoproteins, etc. These were not actual measures of the blood fats themselves but of their carrier chemicals. Thus, for years, for example, it has been known that cholesterol is carried around in the blood by what are known as low density lipoproteins (LDL). Triglycerides, on the other hand, are transported by the group known as very low density lipoproteins (VLDL).

In the mid-1960's the suggestion was made in the medical literature that it was more accurate, in estimating the significance of elevated blood fats in the causation of cardiovascular disease, to measure the lipoprotein rather than the actual levels of cholesterol and triglycerides. This caused a certain amount of consternation and scurrying among medical laboratories because, while the direct determination of cholesterol and triglyceride was a relatively simple procedure, the specific determination of the lipoproteins was quite complex and expensive. Luckily for all concerned, as experience accumulated, the general consensus among medical experts was that no additional information beyond what was learned from a simple cholesterol and triglyceride determination would be gathered by the additional determination of the lipoproteins.

And that was where the situation rested until HDL began to rear its ugly or beautiful head (depending on how one looks at it). What's all the fuss about HDL anyhow? The reasoning is like this: A high cholesterol is bad. But, a high cholesterol is always associated with a high LDL, which, in turn, is also bad. Similarly, with triglyceride, a high triglyceride is none too good. Nor is an elevated VLDL, which is the carrier of triglyceride. HDL, however, turns out to be a peculiar animal in that an elevated HDL seems to be a very important *protector* against cardiovascular disease. Unfortunately, it seems as if we inherit from our ancestors the tendency to have a low or a high HDL level. If that were the only case, then the picture would be quite pessimistic. Some recent articles, however, have pointed out the finding of high HDL levels in, for example, long-distance runners and others who do regular "fitness exercises." Now, if that proves to be true, then there might be something we can all do to increase our HDL levels if the protective effect of HDL is finally proven.

Preliminary reports indicate that cholesterol can be carried not only by LDL but also by HDL, and the higher the HDL cholesterol carrier rate, the less bad is the elevated cholesterol one may find on a pure cholesterol determination. Thus a high cholesterol all of which is carried by LDL is bad. It now seems, however, that a high cholesterol, most of which is carried by HDL, may not be bad at all. Granted that elevated cholesterol is second in pathogenetic importance in causing cardiovascular disease only to elevated blood pressure, then it becomes of great importance to find out if a person has a lot of HDL or LDL. Preliminary long-range reports seem to indicate that the high HDL people do very well from the point of view of cardiovascular morbidity and mortality in spite of elevated cholesterol. If these observations are verified, then, indeed, the HDL story may become one of major importance.

Again, however, a laboratory problem seems to have arisen: How to determine HDL levels? One reads, in the medical literature, of its being a simple test easily added on to the normal cholesterol determination. That would be great, if true! One also reads, in the medical literature, that the test is so complicated that it requires, as a preliminary step, use of a centrifuge as big as a normal size room.

And that's where things stand: HDL may or may not be important. (But it seems to be.) It may or may not be a simple task to determine HDL levels (and this is still being debated); but there is no doubt that it *is* news.

EXERCISE AND THE HEART

A study performed in the late 1960's showed that physically inactive men had a higher incidence of first heart attacks than men who were more active. As a matter of fact, while smokers were shown to have twice as many first coronaries as nonsmokers, no difference was found between the least active nonsmoker and the more active cigarette smokers. Naturally the highest frequency of first coronaries occurred in inactive smokers.

One generally accepted fact is that the first heart attack is lethal to approximately one-half of all men within the first month of onset. This study presented the following results: The least active nonsmoker is nearly twice as likely to experience a rapidly fatal myocardial infarction as the more active cigarette smoker. Inactive men who smoke cigarettes show a mortality experience nearly nine times that of more active nonsmokers of similar age.

Now, none of this is meant to deny the importance of other factors in coronaries such as cholesterol, high blood pressure, diabetes, etc.; rather this study was designed to focus on exercise as a separate factor.

As further medical evidence continues to come in, it appears that the advice that exercise is good for us rests on more and more solid ground. Some persons have always enjoyed exercise—be they calisthenics, competitive sports, or just plain walking—but their advice that others do likewise has often been dismissed as, at best, of no great consequence or, at worst, just based on personal prejudices or preferences.

A nonexerciser who joins the ranks of the exercisers will often report that he feels better, sleeps better, has more regular bowels, and other general nonspecific feelings that one associates with the concept of "increased well-being." And, this is all probably quite true. But, up until now, what answer could one give to the person who says he feels great, sleeps well, has clockwork bowels, and hates to exercise?

Our present answer to this "great-feeling" nonexerciser would go something like this: If you're an American male who has been accustomed to lifelong eating habits of plenty of bacon and eggs, butter, and lots of beef, with good quantities of ice cream and sweets thrown in, *or,* if you've been smoking a pack of cigarettes or more a day for years, *or,* if you've had high blood pressure for sometime now, *or,* if you're a diabetic (even a mild one), *or,* if you've lead a sedentary life associated with relatively constant, even low, levels of stress, *or,* if you used to be always thin or normal weight and have, over the years, become gradually but incontrovertibly overweight, *then,* exercise may very well be *necessary for your heart* to decrease the chances of your dying young from a coronary.

Specifically, what does the *right kind* of exercise do for our heart? (We'll get to which kind is the right kind in a minute.) For one thing regular exercise slows the pulse. Now a slow pulse may not do much for your looks on the beach during the summer, but it can keep you going to the beach a few years longer than if you had a fast pulse. A normal resting pulse is about 72 beats per minute. It is not unusual for a sedentary person to have a resting pulse of 80 to 90. And it is also not unusual for a person who exercises regularly to have a resting pulse in the 60–70 range. Repeated studies have confirmed that, all other factors being equal, the incidence of coronaries is greater in persons with high resting pulses than in those with low resting pulses. Not very dramatic, but real.

A very dramatic finding is what happens to a person when he's had his first coronary after all. As mentioned above, the awful statistics show that, of 100 men who have coronaries, 50–60 of them will be dead within the first month of their coronary attack. *Anything* that will reduce that terrible statistic would be good news. Well, regular exercise is that good news. The death rate in the first month for regular exercisers is less than half of that 50–60% just quoted!

But there's more. Recent studies have shown that regular exercise tends to lower high blood pressure, and it tends to lower elevated cholesterol levels. Both these effects are of great importance since they are, respectively, Public Enemies #1 and #2 on the list of adverse factors that are active in the causation of cardiovascular disease. Anything that subverts their pernicious influence has *got* to be good.

Exercise may have even another effect that may prove to be of great benefit. The heart is supplied by three blood vessels for the nourishment of its own muscle. A "coronary" is usually due to the clogging and eventual closing off of one of these nutrient vessels, so that the heart muscle served by it literally dies from lack of oxygen. Now, if one could somehow get a substitute or a new blood vessel, things might be a lot better. That, however, has proved to be a major stumbling block. It's been only within the past year or so that surgeons have successfully been able to bypass such a blocked or getting-blocked blood vessel by using a substitute vessel which they make out of a vein from somewhere else in the person's body. This is one of the new frontiers of heart surgery, and the procedure itself is not without hazard. However, the heart *can* be stimulated, by regular exercise it seems, to grow microscopic collateral channels for these getting-blocked blood vessels. While these collateral channels are nowhere near as large as the original three blood vessels, they may be able to serve as adequate substitutes if one of the "big three" does close off. Or, if not able to serve as full substitutes, the presence of these collaterals may serve to limit the area of damage to the heart muscle.

So, the right kind of exercise bestows some significant advantages upon the exerciser. What is the right kind of exercise? It turns out that it must be *sustained* exercise for at least 20 minutes three times a week. The sustained exercise must be at what is called a "conditioning pulse rate" (which your physician should be able to help determine for you on an individual basis). Exercise, regardless of how much time it takes, will do your heart no good if your pulse is considerably lower than your own predetermined conditioning pulse rate. And, if you've got as much junk lining the three blood vessels of your heart as most Americans do, exercise at a pulse rate much above your conditioning rate may actually precipitate an episode of coronary oxygen insufficiency—which can be very dangerous.

Now, 20 minutes three times a week may not seem like much, but we must remember that we're talking here about *sustained* exercise, not the kind of wide pulse swings that one experiences in most competitive sports. In these cases, where there are bursts of rapid pulse alternating with brief periods of slowed pulse, the conditioning pulse is *not* sustained, and there is consequently little benefit that accrues to the heart. Recommended exercises include swimming, jogging, running in place, bicycling (stationary or otherwise), and other types where the sustained effort is possible. (Incidentally, isometrics are totally useless from this point of view and may actually be harmful because of the bursts of really high blood pressure they cause.) One measures for the conditioning pulse at the *end* of the exercise period. Take your pulse within the first 15 seconds of cessation of exercise, multiply by the appropriate factor to bring it up to a heart-beats-per-minute reading, and then use this rate to adjust the level of exercise either up or down as necessary to be on the target-conditioning pulse.

That may sound simple, but you'll soon see that it's so much of a workout that it is not advisable to stop your exercise cold at the end of 20 minutes. Rather one should allow a 2–5 minute period of slow tapering off. (Some also recommend an additional 2–5 minute warm-up period before beginning the fully sustained effort.) It is advisable to let at least 2 hours lapse after a meal before beginning to exercise. Finally, it is advised that one take a lukewarm (not hot and not cold) shower 5 to 10 minutes after the end of the exercise period.

So, it's not so simple after all. Is it worth it? After all, it's only *one* factor in coronary prevention. Smoking is bad, high blood pressure is bad, high blood fats are bad. Lack of exercise isn't so bad as any of those three, but it *is* a factor in the total picture—and the total picture involves an important gain or loss: your life.

STRESS TESTING

So popular has the concept of exercising for the sake of cardiovascular fitness become that the question is increasingly raised as to whether or not it really is necessary for all would-be participants to have a medical examination and a stress test prior to their entering their chosen programs.

It should be pointed out that the type of exercise being prescribed is "sub-maximal." Rather than relying on age-height-weight-adjusted tables of "maximal" pulse rates for any one person, it has been suggested that each person's maximum pulse be specifically determined by a carefully monitored, individual test program and that the subsequent level of prescribed exercise be at a pulse level of 5–10 beats per minute below that determined maximum. Current beliefs stress that any exercise significantly below such "sub-maximal" pulse rates will probably be of little or no benefit to the participant. It is chiefly because of this high work-output level required that the recommendation for a preprogram medical screening has been made, to assure that the person is not subjecting himself to excessive and, ultimately, dangerous stress during his chosen program.

The universe of would-be participants may be roughly divided into two groups: those who currently maintain some meaningful level of physical activity and the larger number of those who are, essentially, sedentary. It may very well be "safe" for the former group to make significant increases in their usual exercise levels without the need for a medical "exercise screen." Even for that group, however, there is no assurance that the level so self-chosen really is "sub-maximal" and, therefore, presumably beneficial. Equally, there is always the possibility of moving up to a level that is excessive. For the sedentary group, there is no way of knowing, without a preliminary screening, whether an individual should be indulging in strenuous physical exercise at all, and, if so, at what levels he should be participating.

The American College of Sports Medicine has recently offered a practical subdivision of the universe of sedentary persons. Granting that the achievement of a "recommended" level of exercise will be impossible to determine without a preliminary screening, they suggest an initial breakdown of the group by age. Those persons who are under age 35 and are asymptomatic now and have no histroy of previous cardiovascular disease may enter increased exercise programs if they are not *known* to have any primary coronary heart disease risk factors (hypertension, hyperlipidemia, and cigarette smoking). However, if they have any questions about their current health status, develop symptoms while on their increased programs, or have not had a medical examination during the past 2 years, they should consult with their physician.

For the apparently healthy person who is contemplating an exercise program, the screening examination will not only help to determine a prescribed, specific level of exercise, but it will help unmask any latent arteriosclerotic heart disease that may be present. It is primarily with the latter end in view that a preliminary medical examination and stress test is recommended for all persons over 35 years of age and for those under 35 who do not meet the above criteria. While the degree of complexity of the screen can vary widely, a generally accepted minimum for such an evaluation would include a comprehensive history (with emphasis upon the presence or absence of the usual accepted coronary heart disease risk factors as well as upon specific cardiovascular symptoms) and a complete physical examination (with emphasis not only upon specific signs of cardiopulmonary disease but also upon the presence of conditions which might preclude the performance of the stress test screen in the first place). A baseline 12-lead, resting electrocardiogram (EKG) is another basic minimum screening test, while such blood chemistries as fasting blood glucose, cholesterol, and triglyceride levels, although desirable, are not essential.

The well-known focus of the preliminary screen is the stress test, but it should not be undertaken without the examinations outlined above. The stress test itself is a graded, EKG-monitored exercise test using either a treadmill or a stationary bicycle. Facilities such as an oscilloscope for the continuous monitoring of the EKG before, during, and after the test period are essential. The relatively constant monitoring of pulse and blood pressure is also recommended during the test. The stress test allows for the determiniation of a very specific target pulse for the patient to aim for, one which is, indeed, sub-maximal. By monitoring the various parameters available to the examiner during the stress test, the person's maximal pulse can be relatively easily, and safely, determined. Any significant symptoms of exertional intolerance, such as the development of angina or unusual fatigue or shortness of breath, provide a cut-off point. A fall in blood pressure, onset of nausea, or marked unsteadiness of the patient (among other signs) provide objective cut-off signs and, again, offer a very specific pulse point at which abnormalities begin to manifest themselves. Even significant blood pressure changes (be they a sudden drop or a relatively precipitous rise) or a pulse rate that rises above a predicted maximum, though the level of exertion seems only moderate, should serve to provide a cut-off pulse point. In spite of current belief to the contrary, the actual reason most stress tests have to be terminated prematurely (before some arbitrary "ideal" maximum pulse is attained) is one of the above-listed subjective or objective factors rather than because of an abnormality on the electrocardiogram or oscilloscope-monitor.

After the completion of a screening test as outlined above, an exercise prescription can be recommended that is neither too much nor not enough for the patient and that, by its cardiovascular conditioning effect, may help to avert or ameliorate a cardiovascular catastrophe.

PREVENTION OF CORONARIES

Coronary heart disease is the number 1 killer of Americans today. In spite of the startling and dramatic surgical advances in that area, such as heart transplantation, we still have a long way to go medically in coming up with effective *preventive* measures. (After all, discarding an old heart and substituting a new one for it is scarcely an advance in *preventive* medicine.)

One discouraging factor about the whole problem is that, while we now have a generally good idea of which factors are significant in the causation of coronaries, we don't have final proof that elimination of those factors is successful in prevention. That seeming contradiction can be explained in this way: While the presence of Factors A, B, C, D, E, etc. in a person greatly increases his risk of having a coronary, they may merely be further expressions (rather than causes) of a general underlying tendency to develop a coronary heart attack. In that case, controlling Factors A, B, C, etc in no way alters the basic tendency toward the disease. It would naturally follow that the real reason a person *lacking* Factors A, B, C, etc. isn't likely to develop a coronary is not so much the absence of the factors themselves as that their absence is just a reflection of the more basic absence of a tendency toward coronary atherosclerosis.

If this rather delicate hair-splitting proves to be the true picture, then the whole problem of prevention of coronary heart disease becomes very gloomy indeed, for, to date at least, we have no way of correcting any hereditary basic tendencies. Luckily for us (both doctors and patients) the latest studies are beginning to point in the definite direction that control of certain of the Factors A, B, C, etc. *does* help to prevent the development of coronary atherosclerosis (or, more simply, hardening of the arteries). In such a case it becomes very important to know just what these factors are so that we can institute various measures of control.

A conference of the New York Heart Association pointed out that, among the various factors that doctors have known about for some years now, two are of outstanding importance as predictive elements in the causation of coronaries. The first is hypertension (high blood pressure) and the second is abnormal elevations of various blood fats (such as high cholesterol).

The conclusions regarding hypertension seem fairly firm: controlling blood pressure so that it does not rise above 150 systolic and 100 diastolic seems to be a positive factor in the prevention or the putting off (at least) of a coronary. Besides the classical cutting down on one's salt intake and taking something like phenobarbital, there are many newer blood pressure-controlling medications that can be prescribed so that, by various combinations of drugs, your doctor can bring your pressure down to the ideal of 120/80 if he feels that a drop down to that figure is desirable. In exceptional cases a very specific, surgically remediable cause can be found; in such cases, blood pressure controlling medications are usually not required once the curative surgery has been performed.

The medical profession is currently engaged in performing one big act of faith when it comes to the control of blood fats. While final proof is lacking here that control of abnormal blood lipid elevations actually prevents the development of coronaries, all the advice about diet control that doctors are giving is based on the assumption that such control *is* significant. As a matter of fact, one of the most extensive, organized medical studies ever undertaken in America is the National Diet-Heart Study which is studying the feasibility of preparing, and the general acceptance of, such special diets low in saturated fats (such as fats from meat and dairy products) and high in the preferred unsaturated fats. The attitude of many doctors is that if control of blood fats does prove to be a significant factor in preventing coronaries, their advice to control diet has been all to the good.

Other significant predictive factors in the causation of coronary heart disease are cigarette smoking and diabetes. In the case of the effects of cigarettes on the heart and blood vessels, the value of avoidance of smoking in prevention seems relatively clear. There is no "natural tendency" in the body to react as if it had been smoking and inhaling cigarettes, so whatever adverse effects smoking causes can be completely avoided by not smoking.

The presence of diabetes is a complex factor. Whether it is the diabetes directly, or because diabetics tend to develop high blood pressure and abnormal blood fats which actually are the bad risk factors, is still a matter of controversy. However, it is generally agreed that the control of diabetes by diet, pills, or insulin injections is important to the overall health of the diabetic and, at the very least, is indirectly important to his cardiovascular system.

The problem of obesity remains just that. There still does not seem to be any good scientific evidence that being overweight (in the absence of hypertension, abnormal blood fats, smoking, or diabetes) is a bad thing in itself (unless the obesity is at least 25 to 30% above ideal weight, which is gross obesity indeed and which may then become a significant high-risk factor).

Last, and far from least, is the problem of nervous tension in coronaries. Almost every doctor feels it is a significant factor, but it is almost impossible to study scientifically and, unfortunately, may prove to be the hardest of all to control.

CARDIOPULMONARY RESUSCITATION

There are many occasions where the knowledge of cardiopulmonary resuscitation (CPR) is of vital importance. Most instances where this will prove to be a life-saving measure are for those persons who "drop dead" from a heart attack. Although the likelihood of this catastrophe occurring often, or ever, in the vicinity of any *one* of us is not great, the overall figure for the country as a whole is impressive or depressing—as the case may be. Every year approximately 400,000 Americans die of their heart attacks *before* they can even get to a hospital. Who knows how many of these lives could have been salvaged if someone had been around to apply CPR?

The task falls upon you, the civilian, the nonmedical person. You may feel, "Not me, I don't know anything about it—but if you happen to be the only person around who knows *something* about it you may save a life. Sure, maybe ideally it should be done by a doctor in a hospital setting, but people don't have heart attacks in convenient places. Besides, this life-saving technique is good not only for heart attacks but for any cause of sudden death where the breathing and heartbeat stop, such as in drowning, electric shock, and even those rare cases of sudden collapse when a person is exquisitely allergic to insect stings.

The specific actions that will be outlined may, at first reading, seem confusing and hard to remember—especially if you're only going to be called upon to use them once, or never, in your lifetime—so a brief review of the principles behind them all might help to stick them in your memory. First in importance is that the brain cannot safely go more than 4 or 5 minutes without suffering major, probably irrevocable, damage. In other words, if you're going to get there in time to do any good at all, the catastrophe almost has to happen in your presence so you can get started with CPR immediately.

How do you know that the person hasn't merely fainted? In a true "sudden death" emergency, you will feel no pulse. You can check for this either at the wrist or by feeling in the neck area below the ear at the angle of the jaw. You will also see that the person is not breathing—there is no movement of the chest and you'll not be able to feel any breath coming out from the mouth or nose. The time needed to check for heartbeat and respiration is probably no longer than it took for you to read the preceding two sentences. The final clincher in cases of "sudden death" is the widened, dilated pupils. Push up the person's eyelids: If the pupils are widely dilated, you know the blood supply to the brain has stopped and that you have got to get busy trying to do something about it.

Another set of general principles to keep in mind involve what actually has happened. Why does anyone's heart beat? To supply blood to the body. Why do we need to circulate the blood throughout the body? So that the oxygen which is dissolved in the blood can get to all the vital parts—and one of the most vital (if not *the* most vital) of all organs is the brain. So the main purpose of CPR is to get oxygen to the brain. How do you get it there? By getting oxygen into the lungs where it can dissolve into the blood and then by pumping that blood around by using the patient's own heart to do so. So, the first thing to remember is that you don't start pumping the chest first because whatever blood is pumped has been lying there for a while so that there is very little oxygen left. The first thing you do is breathe oxygen into his lungs. *Then* you pump his chest.

Another general thing to keep in mind is this: The lungs are very large; compared to them, the heart is very small. In order to have an efficient circulation, therefore, you'll need to do less work with the lungs and more with the heart.

Here are the CPR steps: (1) Make sure the airway is clear. Sometimes the tongue has "fallen back" and is causing an obstruction. No need to pull it forward with your fingers. Just do this: Place one hand under his neck and pull up. At the same time place the other hand on his forehead and push back. This will result in the head being tilted down and back on a stretched neck. This will usually open the airway (of course if a foreign object in his mouth—such as slipped dentures—is causing a visible obstruction, it should be removed). (2) Now, as mentioned above: First you get oxygen into his lungs. Your own expired breath is perfectly satisfactory for this purpose. Pinch his nose closed with the hand that is holding back the forehead so that the air you breathe into his mouth will not escape through his nose. Then put your mouth tightly over his and blow until you see his chest rise. Release and repeat four times in order to fill the lungs with air. (3) Pumping the blood through the body is next. Kneeling down at his side, press down on the lower part of his breastbone. The pressure required has to be enough to squeeze out the blood from the heart which is underneath the breastbone. It is always helpful to have the person lying down on a hard, rigid surface so that the heart can be better compressed. Press down using the heel of one hand over the other; keep the elbows stiff as you pump and try for a pumping rate of once a second. Hopefully, someone will be there to help you for this can be very exhausting work otherwise. Thus, one of you pumps the heart, the other does the breathing, and you alternate this every 5 minutes or so. However, if you are alone, you have to return to the lungs every 15 seconds (after 15 compressions, that is) and blow 2–3 big breaths into his lungs before returning down for the next 15 pumpings. Keep up this 15 pumps, 2–3 breath sequence until medical help arrives. It has been pointed out that CPR may result in some broken ribs, but the alternative in a patient who is not breathing is death.

Make sure definitive help is on the way while you are doing all this since the work is very exhausting. You'll know you're saving a life if you see his natural skin color return and especially if his pupils constrict.

You may never need this training, but if the occasion should ever arise, you'll be glad you had it. And so will the patient!

STROKES

Heart trouble is the leading cause of death in the United States; cancer in all its forms takes second place; and strokes are in third place. Although there are many causes for what the layman terms a stroke, the one thing all strokes have in common is major, often catastrophic, damage to a blood vessel in the brain area, with a serious neurological deficit resulting.

One of the causes of this vascular damage is so much build-up of cholesterol-laden deposits along the walls of various blood vessels leading to the brain that, literally, enough nutrient blood can no longer get through because of the blockage. This is what is usually meant when arteriosclerosis is blamed as a cause of a stroke. In other patients, such as those with severe high blood pressure, the impairment in the brain's normal blood supply is not due to the gradually increasing blockage just described, but rather to a massive blowout-type rupture of one of the brain's blood vessels; this is caused by the years of repeated high tension against its walls, with their subsequent weakening and eventual rupture. Other patients have various types of congenital abnormalities of the brain blood vessels which are usually accompanied by serious structural weaknesses of their walls which in turn make them more subject to rupture.

Rarer causes than the above are such things as inflammations of the blood vessel walls, such as from the so-called "collagen diseases," and, perhaps even rarer, the closure of a brain blood vessel by a particle traveling rapidly through the blood stream (be that particle either a blood clot or some foreign substance).

Strokes are really a subdivision of cardiovascular diseases, the main part of which is heart attacks. As such, one would expect them to share the same risk factors. Some of the ones that make a person prone to stroke are high blood pressure (the higher the pressure, the greater the likelihood), diabetes, high blood levels of fats (such as cholesterol), smoking, heart disease, and the use of oral contraceptives.

The mildest of strokes (so mild, indeed, that the layman often does not realize that a true mild stroke has occurred) is the so-called "transient ischemic attack." While no one is sure what causes them, the current thinking is that they represent a brief, nonpermanent, closure of the thickened blood vessel. The importance of transient ischemic attacks is that they often are a harbinger of a more serious stroke yet to come.

The warning signs of transient ischemic attacks include such things as sudden temporary weakness or numbness of part of the body; temporary difficulty with speech; brief change of vision in one eye such as blindness, dimness, or double vision; temporary dizziness or unsteadiness; or even temporary loss of memory. These attacks can be as brief as 2 or 3 minutes, seldom last over a couple of hours, and leave the patient with no permanent neurological alteration. As a matter of fact, the patient usually does not lose consciousness during the transient ischemic attack.

Because it portends a more serious problem, such an attack or series of attacks is often considered sufficient grounds for surgery which can consist of either scraping the occluding material from the involved blood vessel (if that blood vessel is accessible to the surgeon) or the actual cutting out of the affected portion and replacing it with a vascular prosthesis. For those blood vessels which are beyond the surgeon's reach, blood thinners are sometimes used to help prevent recurring attacks or progression to a major stroke.

A major cerebral catastrophe is what most people mean by the term *stroke*. The actual stroke is usually not preceded by preliminary symptoms. When they do occur, however, they usually include dizziness, nausea and vomitting, and transient numbness or weakness of one side of the body. In severest form of a stroke, the patient can suddenly fall to the floor unconscious, partially or completely paralyzed. A peculiarity about strokes is that the patient is most severely afflicted during the first day or two after the onset of the stroke. If the patient can survive those days, there is usually a slow but steady improvement which may last up to 6 months or even a year, so that by the end of that time some patients will have so recovered their normal functions that there will be no neurological deficit remaining.

Specific symptoms of brain damage will be noted depending on which part of the brain is served by the involved blood vessel. Usually the specific symptoms occur on the side of the body opposite to the damaged half of the brain unless the involved blood vessel lies toward the midline of the brain, in which case both sides of the body may be affected. Among the findings one can see are one-side paralysis (hemiplegia), loss of or alteration of sensation of one side of the body, speech disturbances of varying degrees of severity, and sometimes one may even have blindness in one eye. When a person is comatose from a stroke, he may also have an elevated temperature, a rapid pulse, and respirations labored and irregular.

It is impossible to predict who will succumb or who will eventually improve. Thirty-five percent of patients admitted to a hospital with a stroke will die of it. Generally, the older the patient, the worse the prognosis. If the patient really never regains full consciousness, or the ability to speak, or if there seems to be significant mental deterioration, the prognosis is worse.

During the acute period of hospitalization of stroke patients, the medical resources of the hospital and its staff are often called upon to the utmost. A comatose patient, for example, has to have someone to check to make sure that the air passages remain open, someone to make sure that he receives adequate but not too much oxygen, someone to insure that he receives sufficient feedings either through stomach tubes or intravenously to maintain his nutritional and fluid intake, someone to pay careful attention to the usual impaired bladder and bowel functions, and, especially in a patient who will go on to survive but not with complete restoration of his neurological functions, someone to see to it that he does not develop pressure sores on his back from the long periods of lying in bed.

As if all of the above were not enough, the real work with a stroke patient begins when he leaves the hospital. For the person with a permanent weakness or paralysis, not only is the physician follow-up important, but the services of a physiotherapist may be even more important. Others will need a speech therapist. All will need a receptive, involved, and loving family. The latter is not only necessary just to be there physically, but also to supply encouragement to the patient and help to reorient him gradually toward a return to whatever outside world contacts he is able to achieve.

How does one prevent strokes? That's the multimillion dollar question to which so much active research is being devoted in the U.S. The control of high blood pressure is primary, plus anything that can lessen the progression of arteriosclerosis, such as good control of diabetes, of elevated cholesterol levels, and of cigarette smoking. Physical and emotional activities require moderation. Sometimes sedatives are needed to lessen nervousness. Sometimes anticoagulants are of more value in prevention than in treatment, and their use may be considered.

NEW ITEMS IN CARDIOVASCULAR MEDICINE

Unless you're a regular subscriber to the *New England Journal of Medicine,* you probably missed three exciting new pieces of medical information relating to heart attacks that appeared in that journal recently. Fortuitously, one item deals with something that can be done to help prevent getting a heart attack; one deals with the management of most patients during a heart attack; and the third deals with an exciting new concept to apply to patients after they have had their first heart attack.

We all know that cardiovascular disease is the number 1 killer of Americans. Most of us know, by this time, that the single most important risk factor in the causation of cardiovascular disease is hypertension or high blood pressure. The recent study referred to gave statistical significance to an association between hypertension and obesity which had long been suspected by the medical profession and the lay public alike. We all "kind of" knew that if you had high blood pressure and were overweight, it was a good thing to lose weight, but really didn't quite know why that was so. As a matter of fact, even though the medical profession knew this, the main thrust of its advice in the control of blood pressure had been twofold: (1) fairly rigid restrictions of salt from one's diet and (2) the application of various blood pressure-lowering medicines to those patients in whom salt restriction was not sufficient to bring blood pressure levels down to acceptable levels.

The new study shows that a third avenue is now available to the medical approach against high blood pressure: weight reduction. It found statistically significant lowering of blood pressure in any obese hypertensive who lost 10 pounds or more even though salt restriction was specifically excluded as part of the control regimen. While this may not sound like a very exciting discovery, and while it may not be a very popular approach to patients, nonetheless many doctors are so often discouraged by the lack of success in controlling blood pressure in some patients that any real new aid is welcomed.

From the practical standpoint, where does this leave the patient? Salt restriction is by no means thrown out the window. Rather, one more window has been opened: weight loss, to let in some air and light on the problem. The hypertensive who is more than 10 pounds above his ideal weight should consider going to his physician and having an individually planned dietary regimen worked out for him that will succeed in bringing his weight down to better levels. He should continue to watch his salt intake as vigorously as he did before; he should continue to take whatever medicine his doctor prescribed in the same fashion as before; but, the good news is that perhaps after weight loss is achieved, a lowering of medication doses may be a real possibility. For those people whose medication side effects have been a cause of concern, this new approach has to be good news.

The second item concerns the length of stay in the hospital of a person who has experienced a heart attack or coronary. In the Dark Ages when I was in medical school, I remember our professor of medicine saying that if he ever had a coronary, he wanted to be put in bed with whatever clothes he was wearing at the time the episode occurred, heavily sedated, and then left alone for at least 6 weeks. Of course, he was exaggerating, but, just a little. In those days, absolute and prolonged bed rest seemed to be of the utmost urgency during a coronary. As a matter of fact, within the past 15 years I remember a bright young internist on our medical staff coming to me after examining a patient who had come down to the medical department with chest pain. The cardiogram had shown changes of an acute coronary, and arrangements had been made for emergency transportation of the patient to a nearby hospital. I vividly recall the doctor coming into my office, shaking his head, and saying, "He's finished." When I questioned him further, he said that if the patient survived the attack, surely he could never return to work again! And that's the way things were in those days. Prolonged bed rest, long periods of immobility, and then, if the patient was lucky enough to get out of the hospital alive, approximately 6 months of very guarded, very cautious convalescence at home, with many patients never returning to work again— these were standard medical prescriptions.

Things have certainly changed since then in our thinking regarding what to do with coronary patients during their attack. First, probably, was the famous suggestion, by Dr. Levine of Harvard, of getting some coronary patients up in a chair in a few weeks rather than the 6 weeks that used to be practiced. A few years ago, the radical suggestion was made that some patients who had uncomplicated coronaries could actually be sent home within 3 weeks of being admitted to the hospital with their coronary attack, and, now, the latest study comes forth with the incredible suggestion that patients with uncomplicated coronaries can be sent home after 1 week of hospitalization! A follow-up study showed no increase in long-term complications in these patients. Of course, that small percentage of cases of coronaries who have heart failure with their attack or serious disturbances in the heartbeat may not be candidates for such early discharge, but, the majority of coronary cases that make it to the hospital probably would be candidates.

The grim statistics nonetheless remain that over half of coronary attacks are fatal before the patient can even reach the hospital. The problem is still a dreadful one for Americans, and prevention is still of the utmost importance. Nobody wants to have a coronary, but this new approach removes the cloud of chronic invalidism that unnecessarily hung over so many coronary patients. They can get back to their own life-style sooner; they can get back to work sooner; their self-confidence and self-esteem cannot help but be improved by this early resumption of normal life activities.

The third report concerned a new and exciting approach to a patient who has had a coronary. A little less than a month after the attack, a large series of patients was put on a gout-controlling drug that has been around the medical scene for almost 20 years. Why a drug that works in gout should have diminished the frequency of sudden deaths after the first heart attack is anybody's guess. It's a combination of serendipity and medical insight. At any rate, the preliminary conclusions, which are being currently widely tested to assure their ultimate validity, indicated that patients on this medication experienced only half as many episodes of sudden death as those who were put on no medication or a sham medication. Sure, this medication has some side effects: it can cause blood count problems in some few patients, it can aggravate acid stomachs and ulcers, some people might even get a rash, but, if it proves out that this medicine has succeeded in reducing sudden deaths after the first coronary by 50% or more, it will prove to have been one of the most dramatic medical discoveries of the past 10–20 years.

HEMORRHOIDS

For a condition that is benign, hemorrhoids are responsible for an awful lot of discomfort and, in some people, for a lot of worry. "An awful lot of discomfort" because piles (which is the common name for hemorrhoids) are very common; and, "an awful lot of worry" because rectal bleeding, which is the most common manifestation of hemorrhoids, has been widely advertised as one of the early manifestations of rectal cancer.

Far from being cancer or even a precancerous condition, hemorrhoids are merely another case of varicose veins. This basic distended-vein cause is the same regardless of whether a person suffers from internal or external hemorrhoids. The only difference between the two diagnoses is that internal hemorrhoids are located higher up in the rectal canal than external hemorrhoids.

While rectal bleeding can be an early sign of colon cancer, once the bleeding is established to be of hemorrhoidal origin, the patient can be reassured that this is in no way connected with a cancerous condition. In contrast to suspicious rectal bleeding which, while it is usually bright red, can sometimes be darker and is often found mixed in with the stool substance itself, hemorrhoidal bleeding is always bright red and, if it appears on the stool at all, is always located as a slight spotty superficial coating of the stool surface itself. Hemorrhoidal bleeding surely is the chief cause of blood-flecking of the toilet tissue; and also, especially in those cases where the rupture of a relatively large hemorrhoidal vessel occurs, the chief cause of blood staining the water in the toilet bowl.

Internal hemorrhoids usually bleed. If they are greatly congested, they can give the patient a suggestion of local rectal fullness. While they can cause itching and can also protrude through the anal opening, these two occurrences are much less common with internal than with external hemorrhoids. The latter not only can bleed and give a sense of fullness but quite often can cause itching. And it is the external hemorrhoid which is the more likely to cause that extremely painful complication of hemorrhoids: thrombosis and prolapse.

Where the usual hemorrhoidal bleeding will stop in a few minutes and heal over in a day or so, the rarer occurrences of thrombosis and/or prolapse will incapacitate, or at least greatly bother, the afflicted patient for a week or so. Many a patient who is subjected to this more painful complication has noticed that his hemorrhoidal attack may not be preceded or accompanied by rectal bleeding at all. These hemorrhoidal inflammations result in so much pressure and congestion that the blood in the involved vein actually clots; and it is that swollen, clotted vein which, having little space to expand within the relatively narrow confines of the anal canal, protrudes and prolapses downward and outward to form the inflamed visible manifestation of a thrombosed hemorrhoid.

What causes hemorrhoids? No one knows, but among the chief factors is heredity. Increased intra-abdominal pressure, such as occurs in pregnancy, abdominal tumors, liver disease, or even obesity can be responsible. One such increase in pressure is the obvious case of straining at stool. The kind of straining at stool because of a hard dry stool can be remedied by advising the hemorrhoid sufferer to drink lots of fluids and to increase the bulk content of his stool either by increasing his dietary intake of roughage in the form of raw fruits and vegetables, or, if that is not sufficient, by adding to his daily intake a bulky stool softener, such as Metamucil. The other kind of straining at stool that is to be avoided occurs in those people who feel that they must have a daily bowel movement at a set time, regardless of the fullness of their lower rectal canal. Surely, this kind of compulsiveness should be discouraged. Having a bowel movement when nature calls is fine; trying to force a bowel movement when nature is silent is foolish—and can lead to, or aggravate, hemorrhoids.

After bowel movements, hemorrhoid sufferers should cleanse the area with moist tissue by patting rather than rubbing. If at all possible, a mild soap washing followed by adequate tissue rinsing of the area is an excellent preventive of hemorrhoidal episodes.

Once the hemorrhoid is thrombosed and protruding, however, little can be done other than to grin and bear it. Hot baths, bed rest, and pain medications may be required for the 4 or 5 days during which the episode lasts.

Surgery should be a last resort not only because it is often unnecessary if one conscientiously follows the above recommendations, but especially because hemorrhoids can return after surgery. Some years ago injection treatments of irritating chemicals were used in an attempt to scar down the involved blood vessels, but they are used much less frequently nowadays. Recently, a not-painless but relatively effective method of treating hemorrhoids has been to put a rubber band around them and "strangulate them off" (for some patients, however, that particular cure sounds worse than the disease).

4
Dental

CAVITIES

Two of the chief problems that teeth are heir to are cavities and pyorrhea—both quite prevalent, both quite preventable.

Cavities, of course, are diseases of the teeth themselves: what is usually referred to as tooth decay. Pyorrhea is the result of disease in the gums and supporting structures: what is often called periodontal disease. The former can occur at all ages—but especially in our younger years; the latter occurs mostly in older persons.

Dental caries (as cavities are more technically called) have been estimated to affect 98% of our population. It has been estimated that tooth decay attacks three of the average child's teeth by the time he reaches school age. The average 15 year old has been estimated to have 11 teeth afflicted by cavities.

What causes cavities? Many things do, among which three are probably the most important. First, there must be sufficient quantities of the right bacteria living in the mouth. No single agent is responsible; rather a combination of acid-producing bacteria is required to increase the acidity in the immediate vicinity of the external surface of the tooth (which is where all cavities begin; they do not start on the inside and work their way out).

The second requirement for cavities is the right food for these bacteria to thrive on. Most of it is supplied by the sugar and starches in the food we eat. The more often one eats, the more active his bacteria are. It is actually the acid wastes of bacterial digestion and fermentation that go on to dissolve tooth enamel. The frequency with which starches are consumed is more important than the total quantity consumed. This is why between-meal carbohydrate snacks are the worst offenders. The consistency of the ingested carbohydrate is also important (the stickier the food, the longer it takes to be cleared completely from the mouth and thus the more damage it can cause). Of course, if one brushed the teeth immediately following eating, this would be effective both in removing residual food products and also in minimizing the effect of bacterial action.

Finally, we have an important, but indefinable, factor: the inherent susceptibility of the teeth to these acids. Some people just seem to inherit strong teeth that rarely, if ever, get cavities. Lucky for them. Their luck, however, does not hold for the overwhelming majority of us. One example of susceptibility to cavities that stems from the person himself is something as simple as the natural amount of his saliva flow—diminished flow being associated with an increased susceptibility to cavities.

What can be done about cavities? Hopefully, by now, the "Great Fluoride Controversy" has subsided so that we can see the whites of their teeth through the subsiding smoke and haze. There really is, I believe, overwhelming evidence that fluoride is an important element in helping to prevent tooth decay. Even when fluoride is present in such minute quantities as one unit of fluoride in 1 million units of water, the tooth decay rate falls by about 60%.

For those people who do not have the advantage of fluoridated water, there are various methods by which fluoride can be helpfully utilized. One way that can be arranged through a dentist is the direct application of fluoride to the teeth for a few minutes a day by means of a very thick semi-solution held close by a plastic mouthpiece. It can also be given daily with vitamins. This latter method is especially important for young children living in nonfluoridated water areas. It has been suggested that they take *daily* fluorides (with or without their vitamins) from birth until at least after their permanent teeth have erupted. A safe age would be up to their 10th year. Another way fluoride can be ingested is by having it added to salt just the way iodine is to iodized salt.

A new, exciting approach to the cavity problem has recently gained prominence. It's based on the old idea of keeping bacteria out of nesting places in the small cracks and pits on the chewing surfaces of the teeth. In the past some dentists filled the larger cracks, or ground the surfaces slightly to smooth out irregularities, in order to minimize decay on these surfaces. The new development is a durable, but still experimental, plastic sealant. It is hoped that, when the paint is put on after the teeth are thoroughly cleaned, it will last for 2 or more years.

Since it is unlikely that people will stop eating sweets, one further research suggestion to them has been the use of specific additives to counteract decay—but this is far from any immediate realization.

Meanwhile, as the research goes on, what do we do about it? Remember: destruction of your teeth and gums doesn't happen overnight. So the sooner you take proper preventive action, the better the chance for continued good dental health.

PYORRHEA

The second major problem of the oral cavity is pyorrhea and other periodontal disease. Periodontal disease means, generally, disease of the gums and supporting structures of the teeth. Whereas cavities tend to occur especially often in the earlier years of life, periodontal disease, on the other hand, tends to occur toward the other end of the age spectrum. Thus, it afflicts two out of three middle-aged Americans. It has been estimated that destruction of the tissues and structures that hold teeth fast in their sockets accounts for 75% of tooth loss after the age of 40. In spite of these rather impressive figures, it seems as if the American public isn't too impressed. Some depressing figures reported by dentists reveal that fewer than 5% of their dental visits are for gum treatments.

The bad thing about periodontal disease is that it can result in an insidious loss of perfectly sound teeth. It does this not by direct attack like tooth decay but rather by undermining the supporting structures, which results in loosening of the teeth. Usually it begins as a reddening and swelling of the gums. This gingivitis may be accompanied by occasional bleeding, but, nonetheless, this is still an easily reversible stage. However, if the inflammation is allowed to progress, pockets are created between the gums and the teeth in which germs and food particles can lodge. They tend to further the inflammation, pushing the gums further away from the teeth as the pockets deepen. When pus has formed in these pockets, the condition is known as pyorrhea. At this stage the infected gums can ulcerate and bleed and usually are painful. In the final stage, there is destruction of the supporting structures and bone which anchor the teeth and, eventually, the loosened teeth fall out.

It has been estimated that 67 million Americans have periodontal disease and that there are 20 million adults who have lost all their teeth because of it! Although the full-blown condition is usually not noticed until after age 30, it has been estimated that four out of five mid-teenagers have gingivitis which is the easily reversible form of the disease. One argument for starting preventive measures early is that 4% of these mid-teenagers actually had an advanced stage.

The chief causes of periodontal disease are bacteria, tartar, and food debris. Thus, when soft particles of food remain on the teeth, bacteria thrive. Soon, sticky masses of bacteria and their waste products form films called plaque. These can be removed by thorough cleaning daily by brushing and by the use of dental floss or tape and water sprays or jets.

If neglected, plaque will harden within 2–14 days into a crustlike material called calculus or tartar. Home care cannot, however, remove tartar. Here, regular interval cleaning by a dentist is needed.

It used to be believed that the mechanical separation of gums from teeth by wedges of calculus was the chief irritant in gum inflammation. Now it is felt that the living, nonmineralized bacterial layer at the junction between gums and teeth causes most of the damage.

Other factors operative in periodontal disease include advancing age, poor alignment of the teeth, missing teeth (which often causes others to drift out of position), and the habit of grinding the teeth. Gum irritation caused by worn fillings, sharp edges of decayed teeth, and ill-fitting dentures is another contributing factor. Some less frequent factors include mouth breathing, lip biting, and an unusual amount of tongue pressing against the teeth. Finally, poor nutrition including protein, mineral, and vitamin deficiency is also implicated.

Periodontal disease is more likely to occur and be more severe among persons with various systemic disorders, such as diabetes and chronic vascular disease. Smoking also is a contributing factor. The hormonal changes associated with pregnancy and the menopause, family history, and emotional stress have also been considered by some scientists as important predisposing or contributing factors.

What can be done? Early detection and dedicated home care are the key concepts. Good oral hygiene remains the one most effective preventive measure. Careful daily brushing will stimulate the circulation in gum tissue and remove bacterial plaques. The regular removal of tartar, every 6 months or so, by your dentist plus occasional X-rays for the detection of bone damage are also important. Sometimes the replacement of missing teeth or even "bite" correction is necessary.

Once periodontal disease has gotten started, treatment will depend on the stage of the disease. If it has not progressed far, it may only be necessary to remove soft bacteria deposits and tartar from around and under the gums. If pockets have formed between the teeth and gums, often they must be surgically treated. In its final stage, when periodontal disease attacks the bone which supports the teeth, treatment may require bone and reconstructive surgery.

5
Dermatology

ACNE

Medical conditions often cause misery, but one of the conditions that has probably been responsible for more misery than a host of other conditions put together isn't even serious enough to be labeled an illness. The condition in question is acne, and I suspect that many an acne sufferer would gladly settle for a quick 3-week bout of pneumonia in exchange for the awkward, embarrassed, unhappy "years of the pimples."

Acne is, as at least 80% of us have learned during our adolescence or early adulthood, a skin disease or condition that affects primarily the face and neck but that can also involve the chest and back. Not only is it not fatal, but it really doesn't make you sick when you have it. But in some persons (luckily in the minority) it can become very severe and extensive even though they *don't* feel physically ill. Their acne may cause so much scarring and widespread involvement and secondary localized infections that it may persist into middle age.

It begins with the lowly blackhead which is just a skin pore blocked by skin oils and shed skin cells. Incidentally, the dark upper portion of superficial blackheads is not usually caused by dirt but rather is secondary to chemical changes in the pore-blocking material. And then, of course, there are deeper "blackheads" which really do not reach the surface. In some persons their acne never progresses beyond this stage.

The second stage has not only blackheads but also inflammation around the blocked pores along with small *superficial* pus pimples. It is important to know that this stage, which is usually confined to the face, will not produce significant scarring *unless the lesions are scratched and picked.* This form can subside in 1 or 2 years with appropriate treatment.

The third stage has, along with second stage findings, a tendency toward *deeper* areas of inflammation. Part of what has happened is that the blocked pores have ruptured inwardly, part is that bacteria have settled in these inflamed areas, causing deep pockets of infection. This is the type often found not only on the face but also on the neck, upper shoulder, and upper chest. This is the critical stage during which significant scarring can occur both to the skin and to the soul.

Finally we have, in the last stage, what is called infected cystic acne. Here the subsurface infections can actually join together, causing small canals and pockets of pus under the skin. This type can even spread up toward the scalp and is quite often associated with scars and cordlike skin bulges once the lesions begin to quiet down. Patients suffering from stage 4 acne can actually have pain in the involved areas.

The causes of all this mess and misery are many factors, chief of which are probably heredity and hormones. One often finds family histories of acne of varying degrees of severity in other members of the patient's family. But this is not enough for, the strongest family history notwithstanding, if the hormonal changes of puberty did not occur, then there would be no resultant acne.

Many persons may not realize that men make both male and female sex hormones and that females make both female and male sex hormones. Acne turns out to be one of the hormonal common meeting grounds because the significant acne hormone, in both sexes, is the male hormone. (This, of course, does not mean that there will be evidence of masculinization in afflicted females.)

Certain foods or medicines can aggravate acne in some patients. Especially to be avoided are chocolate, nuts (including peanut butter), and cola drinks. Shellfish may also be an offender and are best avoided in serious cases. Medicines containing bromides or iodides should also be avoided. Scratching, picking, or other trauma to the skin can also aggravate acne, as can climate changes. Acne will often flare in the winter and, paradoxically, also in excessively hot, humid weather. Many girls notice flareups around the time of their periods. Occasionally (although this is relatively unusual in persons eating balanced diets), vitamin A deficiency may be a factor. Finally, acne can flare during periods of psychological stress.

What can one do about it? As one medical text put it, "The treatment of acne has possibly received as much attention as any problem in all of medicine, both in lay and scientific journals. The multiplicity of methods bespeaks the absence of any single effective and specific therapy."

Among the general measures used are: wash the involved areas twice a day with a good toilet soap or one containing such antibacterial agents as hexacholorophene. A soft complexion brush or abrasive brush is to be avoided when the lesions are inflamed. Blackheads may, with careful extraction with a special extractor, be removed once or twice a week after a preliminary 10–15 minutes of warm towel soaks.

Do not pick crusts. There are available, through a doctor's prescription, lotions which can help unplug pores and cause mild peeling away of superficial blocked-skin layers. Occasionally a doctor may prescribe a cream containing antibiotics with or without added cortisone.

For stage 3 and 4 acne there is the administration of antibiotics—small doses for weeks or even months. These should always be taken under a doctor's guidance. Finally, all stages probably benefit from a warm sunny climate with absence of high heat and humidity. The great majority of acne sufferers will find relief as they leave their adolescent years.

ATHLETE'S FOOT

Many of us experience a flare-up of a common, annoying, but absolutely nonfatal condition called athlete's foot. So common is this condition that it has been estimated that over half of the adult population has ringworm of the feet at sometime during their lives.

Many of us don't realize that athlete's foot is ringworm, although many people think of it as an infection of *some* sort. As ringworm, however, it shares many of its peculiar infectivity characteristics.

Thus, it is not absolutely infectious. For example, almost everyone who has ever been exposed to the measles or chickenpox virus will get those diseases because those two viruses have almost absolute infectivity. This type of infectivity is not true for ringworm infections. Some people just don't ever get them even though they are exposed to the same environmental circumstances at the same time when someone else *will* get them.

A number of factors are important in the acquisition and severity of this disorder. Heredity, of all things, seems to be a most important factor even though it's very hard to pin down what this means. Certainly, there is no question of hereditary transmission of athlete's foot. That just doesn't happen! Many a mysterious theory has been offered as an explanation for the hereditary factor: the sweat may be too acid; the sweat is not acid enough; the skin is thicker and so has greater resistance; no, the skin is thinner and so has less resistance because the circulation is deeper under the skin, etc. Two of the suggestions that probably are valid have to do with sweating and the body's resistance factors. It may very well be that some people's feet are heavily bathed in perspiration regularly, and such a condition "may run in families." Certainly, the immunological or resistance factors that a person has are in great part due to his hereditary makeup.

There may also be hormonal factors operative in athlete's foot. Children certainly go around barefoot more often and in stranger places than the majority of adults; and yet athlete's foot is rarely, if ever, seen in children. It's an adult disease. Another genetic factor to be considered is that men get athlete's foot more commonly than women. Of course, this has nothing to do with the fact that there are more men athletes than women athletes, since the condition is by no means exclusively one of athletes.

Added to whatever internal factors there may be is, of course, a set of necessary external factors. The dry foot just *doesn't* seem to get athlete's foot. Even the person with the heaviest perspiration of his feet will have a dry foot if he goes barefoot. Whatever else is operative on the local environmental level, moisture may be important in letting the infection catch hold. Thus, a person who has had it once before and who wants to avoid flareups, or a person who seems to fit the description of those whose feet are fertile ground for athlete's foot should try to wear things like cotton socks or, in the winter, wool (if necessary) because they are absorbent. Leather shoes are much to be preferred to the new plastic "leather" since the latter doesn't "breathe."

Foot hygiene is important in that, after bathing, the feet must be dried very carefully and thoroughly, including the individual areas between the toes. A bland dusting powder is often helpful to get the feet dry.

The condition manifests itself in at least three ways. Perhaps the most annoying, because it is so itchy, is a kind of eruption of little blistery pimples that can occur around the foot, on the instep, or on the bottom. As these lesions heal, they dry and scale off and may become brownish, making it look as if there were a little blood under the skin. Some people get just this form, and when it recurs, it recurs in just this form. One of the most peculiar reactions in all of medicine is associated with this blistery, pimply, itchy type of athlete's foot. This is known as the "id" reaction (abbreviation for dermatophytid). What happens in an id reaction is that these same blistery pimples that are occurring on the feet will occur on the fingers, between the fingers, and on the hands themselves. Often they serve as a clue to the doctor for the presence of a flareup of athlete's foot of the feet even though the patient may not be aware of the latter. Interestingly enough, while it is possible to culture the invading fungus from the foot lesions, it is not possible to culture the lesions of the hands because they are almost invariably sterile. No organisms are present even though they look like the condition of the feet. What we think happens is that an allergic reaction takes place in the body to the presence of the invading fungus of the feet, and that allergic reaction manifests itself on the hands. Of course, the hand rash, being free of organisms, is not infectious. Many a patient will be surprised when the suggestion is made that the treatment be directed towards his feet rather than his hands because, generally, with the clearing up or subsidence of the foot infection, the hand reaction clears spontaneously.

The second form of athlete's foot, which is probably what most people mean by athlete's foot, is cracking or scaling or fissuring between the toes. A certain amount of maceration of the skin also is present. This form may also have the above id reaction of the hands. In this case, the id reaction is as above (blistery pimples), while the feet may have no blisters or pimples but rather the cracks and fissuring. While annoying, and often persistent, this form is not so itchy as the first form.

The third form is the chronic, scaling, thickening of the skin which is usually seen over the heel or other plantar surfaces of the foot. This form is often associated with a fungus infection of the toenails. The nails become thick and lusterless with an accumulation of debris under the toenails which, at times, becomes so large and thick that the nail plate actually becomes separated and the nail may be destroyed. This form is the most difficult of all the forms to eradicate.

I hope that the above descriptions have been lurid enough to convince you that, even though you are not going to die of athlete's foot, this is a condition for which you should see your doctor. Early treatment may prevent or at least forestall progression into the more chronic stages. The few brief hints that follow aren't meant in any way to suggest that this is the entire treatment, or that they can be used instead of seeing your doctor.

In the acute blistery pimply form, warm soaks to the foot or compresses of mild salt solution applied to the foot two or three times a day can be helpful. The application of a 1% to 2% aqueous solution of mercurochrome right after the soaks or compresses is a good idea. No greasy preparation should be applied. Some dermatologists recommend hot diluted potassium permanganate solutions. This is the famous medicine that makes the feet purple (temporarily). In the more chronic conditions, especially when you have considerable thickening of the toenails and the heels of the foot, a prescription medicine, griseofulvin, may be used but *only under a doctor's careful prescription.* For one thing, this is not a magic medicine. It usually takes a long time, up to 6 or more months, to be completely successful; and in a number of cases, it doesn't work even then. Secondly, this is a systemic medication since it has to be taken by mouth. Thirdly, this is a powerful medicine and has side effects. Even though the side effects are relatively uncommon, blood changes, kidney disorders, liver disorders, diarrhea, and skin disorders can occur.

There are other forms of medications available for the condition, but all treatment should be under your doctor's supervision.

BALDNESS

This topic is dear to my heart (or, should I say, head?). It's what many a young man worries about, it's what many an older man has to learn to live with, and it's something almost all women dread: baldness.

Naturally, baldness is much more common in men than in women. In both sexes, however, the commonest cause of hair loss is heredity —which is, in most cases, another way of saying you can't do anything about it. In the overwhelming majority of cases, hereditary baldness is permanent and is caused by actual disappearance of the hair roots and dying out of the hair follicles which are the shells of tissue surrounding the hair root and from which it grows and derives its nourishment.

In most persons, their "hair history" is related to their body growth, sexual development, and aging. For example, body growth effects can be seen in the fact that one never sees baldness in a young boy who may later go on to develop typical male baldness. Sexual development effects are seen in the fact that men who, by accident, surgery, disease, or defects of some congenital form or other, never have true development of their testicles and the normal sex hormones that are secreted by them, do not become bald, regardless of any hereditary tendency they may have. You need, therefore, for typical male baldness, body development and normal sexual maturation. Much as I hate to do it, I think one myth that should finally be laid to rest is that the man who is bald is more virile than the man who has a normal head of hair. The bald man's sex hormones are not higher than anyone else's; all that happens is that, when his sex hormones reach normal levels, they serve to trigger his baldness which, basically, is hereditary.

Aging is a factor in hair loss in that, in aging, hair follicles generally become smaller and some disappear. The smaller the follicles, the finer and shorter the hair. Most men who are becoming bald have a lot of fine short hair that will never grow thicker or longer because of the smaller size of their follicles and also because their hair growth cycle is usually shorter than average: lasting from 3–6 months rather than the more normal 2–3 years.

These underlying factors in baldness are true for both sexes except that, usually, the hair loss in women is not so severe as in men. For one thing, women make significantly fewer quantities of male hormones than men do; for another, estrogen (which is the chief female sex hormone) actually has a protective action against baldness. But the factor of aging, in women, combines increase in years with decrease in protective female hormones so that there can be some hair loss.

What are some of the more uncommon causes of hair loss? For example, some people will complain of a sudden widespread thinning of the hair. In such cases, there may have been a significant generalized body illness or event 3 or 4 months prior to the hair loss; such events as childbirth, surgery, or a high fever may have been the culprit. Usually the hair regrows normally in such cases.

At times, an underlying disorder of the internal (though nonsexual) organs may be to blame. Underactive thyroid is often associated with coarse, thin hair, while very soft, fine hair may be seen in overactivity of the thyroid. Abnormally low functioning of the pituitary gland in the brain can also be associated with fine, dry, thinning head hair. A good clue to such a condition is the loss of hair in the outer third of the eyebrows, and also there is often a concomitant loss of body hair.

Sometimes, certain medicines can cause loss of hair. In some persons anticoagulants (or "blood thinners" as they are often popularly called) can cause loss of hair. Also some of the newer anticancer drugs can cause a rapid loss of hair. Usually the hair will grow back when the agent is stopped.

Besides some of the above-listed modern drugs as a cause of hair loss, some of the modern grooming habits are being more and more implicated. Some dermatologists feel that back-combing (teasing) or using rollers and curlers that produce undue traction on the hair roots are the commonest current explanation for localized hair loss in women. Permanent waves and hair dyes also can damage the hair shaft and break off the hair. Usually, in these instances, the hair will regrow; but repeated undue traction may lead to irreversible loss. When hair straightening was more popular among blacks than it is now, hot combs used in straightening the hair often caused severe traction with subsequent hair loss.

Sometimes the loss of hair is due to scarring of the hair follicles which can follow exposure to high doses of X-rays (such as are used not so much in diagnostic X-rays as in X-rays for treatment of various conditions such as cancer). Scarring can also follow burns from heat and even chemical burns. Some generalized systemic diseases can also cause scarring. Examples include lupus erythematosus, advanced syphilis, and deep bacterial or fungus infections. Since the hair follicles are destroyed by scarring, such hair loss is permanent.

There is a condition of patchy baldness called alopecia areata. While in children the cause is assumed to be ringworm, the condition may develop in a patient at any age. Surprisingly, these persons are usually high-strung and nervous. At times, the patient is under stress in his personal or business life, lending further support to the theory that this condition may have some significant psychogenic causative factors.

One of the weirdest of all forms of hair loss is called trichotillomania, which is one of the fanciest of all medical names for a compulsion to pull one's hair out. Sometimes the patient isn't even aware of his pulling and tugging at one spot of hair until others point it out to him. Unfortunately, in alopecia areata and trichotillomania, the hair may not always grow back.

DANDRUFF

An attractive young girl once asked me how often she should apply lanolin to a scaling patch of dandruff that she'd had in her scalp for months.

"Lanolin? You don't want to use that; that's greasy."

"Of course it's oily, but that's just what I want to do: restore my skins oils to get rid of the dandruff. You see, I have dry skin which, of course, is why I have dandruff."

"Dry skin? You have oily skin—that's what causes dandruff. Lanolin will only makes things oilier."

At that point she looked at me as if I were kidding her. Finally, with the use of some dermatology textbooks, and pictures, and articles, I was able to convince her. Her final suggestion was, "Why don't you write about that? Lots of people think dandruff is caused by dry skin."

So, for those who still believe otherwise, let me state that dandruff occurs only from oily skins. As a simple but final proof, press some dandruff scales between two pieces of tissue paper. By doing this, you are pressing the oiliness out of the scales, leaving the grease mark on the tissue.

Dandruff is really only one symptom of a more extensive skin condition known as seborrheic dermatitis. Basically, the latter is a chronic, reddish, scaling skin condition. It may or may not be associated with an actual skin inflammation; it is often associated with an acne condition or, at least, an acne tendency. All of this needs an increase in skin oils before it can develop. That's one of the reasons these conditions are not seen before puberty.

There are sweat glands and there are oil glands in the skin. The former are distributed all over the body and function from early infancy. The latter are usually located along the side of or at the base of hair follicles but do not really begin functioning until about the time of puberty. Their function seems to be related to the secretion of sex hormones, because those persons who, for whatever reason, lack the normal amounts of sex hormones do not develop oily skins, acne, seborrheic dermatitis, or dandruff regardless of how old they are.

As was mentioned in the article on acne, both sexes secrete male and female hormones. It seems that it is the male hormone that is especially active in oily skin conditions. This does not, of course, mean that there is anything wrong with a girl who has dandruff and acne. What is probably going on is an unusual, perhaps inherited, sensitivity of her skin to the effect of such hormones or some temporary imbalance between the male and female hormones.

It is this hormonal relationship that is probably responsible for one of the common misconceptions about dandruff. Many a young man has frantically tried to get rid of his dandruff condition for fear it would lead to baldness. Dandruff, oily skin, seborrheic dermatitis—whatever label you use—does not lead to baldness. Baldness is caused by male sex hormones in someone who usually has a hereditary predisposition to it in the first place. If such a person never developed any male hormones, regardless of his heredity, he'd never become bald. So both dandruff and baldness can be seen as due to a common cause: male sex hormone.

The dandruff picture is not simply a hormonal one, however, because, although the condition is more prevalent in men than women, it does occur in the latter. It's more common in brown-eyed people—and that has nothing to do with sex hormones. And it's more common in brunettes—and that has nothing to do with sex hormones.

The redness and scaling that go along with dandruff are not necessarily limited to the scalp but can occur either in other hairy areas or in those few nonhairy body areas which are rich in oil glands. Thus, it can occur behind the ears, behind the jaw, at the eyebrows and eyelids, along the sides of the nose, in the ear canals, in the center of the chest and/or upper back, in the armpits, around the navel, and in the groin. Notable exceptions to the above are that dandruff is rarely seen on the arms and legs themselves regardless of the amount of hair covering them.

The condition cannot be cured because it really isn't a disease in the usual sense. Certainly it is not infectious or contagious. It does tend to flare and subside naturally or as a result of treatment. It will ordinarily improve during the summer months, unless the weather is very hot and humid. There are even reported cases in which it has flared subsequent to periods of tension or even loss of sleep. Exposure to natural sunlight is almost always helpful.

For a mild dandruff condition of the scalp, often all that is required is more frequent shampooing. If, however, the scales recur rapidly (within 2 or 3 days), then there is a large variety of special shampoos available. It is best, however, to check with the family physician; for example, one of the most remarkably effective of all dandruff controllers is available by prescription only.

MOLES AND KERATOSES

"Skin Tumor" sounds like an ominous diagnosis, and yet in the great majority of cases such lesions are almost always benign. As a matter of fact, there are probably very few adults who do not have skin tumors of some kind. The misconception arises because most people think that "tumor" means "cancer" when, instead, all it means is swelling.

Perhaps the most common benign skin tumor is a seborrheic keratosis. It can occur virtually anywhere on the body, in parts that may or may not be exposed to the sun, which is often helpful in distinguishing it from the more serious senile or actinic keratosis. Even though they can occur anywhere, seborrheic keratoses are especially common on the trunk, arms, neck, and scalp. They are quite unusual below the hip area.

Although, eventually, they have a typical brownish-grayish-blackish greasy, warty appearance, seborrheic keratoses ordinarily start as a slight yellowish or brownish, somewhat scaly, small area of the skin which, even in its early stages, feels greasy. One of the most apt descriptions of an early seborrheic keratosis is that it resembles a drop of a rather dirty candle wax on the skin.

These seborrheic keratoses are often multiple, enlarge slowly, and are rarely larger than 1/2" in their longest diameters. Not infrequently, pieces of lesions or the whole of such a lesion may fall off, only to recur in a few weeks or months. The important thing to remember about these is that they are benign and require no treatment from a medical standpoint. Some people prefer to have them removed for cosmetic purposes. This removal is usually not a major procedure.

The second large category of keratoses is senile or actinic keratosis (actinic means exposure to the sun's rays). Although such lesions can occur with aging, the great majority of them are precipitated by years of exposure to sunlight. This is why they are usually seen in the forearm or hand area and on the forehead or neck. Rarely, if ever, are they seen in places which are covered by clothing.

These, also, are brownish or grayish raised lesions when first developed; but they always lack that peculiar appearance and greasy feel of the seborrheic keratosis. Quite often senile keratoses have a gritty, horny, roughly irregular, scratchy feel to them that further serves to distinguish them from seborrheic keratoses.

It should be emphasized that senile keratoses are not cancerous lesions. Even though most dermatologists recommend their removal, it is not so much because of the lesions themselves as because of their potential for becoming malignant. It is hard to give an exact figure, but it is probable that far fewer than half of such lesions would become malignant if left alone. However, wisely, dermatologists do not play the percentage game when it comes to a true actinic keratosis. They recommend removal which is usually as simple as that for a seborrheic keratosis.

Even in those few cases which have not been removed and have developed a true cancer, the type of cancer which develops is quite often of a low grade of malignancy and therefore is associated with a very high cure rate. These skin cancers are called squamous-cell epitheliomas; if they are neglected, they can spread elsewhere in the body.

There is another type of skin cancer which is very unusual in its behavior from cancers in general. It is called a basal-cell epithelioma, and in contrast to all other body cancers, it does not spread to other parts of the body even if neglected. However, basal-cell epitheliomas can get very large, and they can erode the underlying skin and, even, bones. So, even when it comes to true skin cancers, the squamous-cell type is of low malignancy and the basal-cell type does not spread at all.

There is, however, one dreaded form of skin cancer which can spread even though the original skin lesion looks small and relatively nonexciting. The type we are referring to here is malignant melanoma. Usually occurring on exposed surfaces of the body, these often look like flat, large freckles. Often they have scattered black nodules on their surface, and they frequently go through a peculiar rainbow of colors as they grow. They can be bluish or reddish or purplish, even an opalescent blue-gray, and, sometimes, even white. These are the notorious skin lesions one is warned about when we read of the changing size or color of skin moles as a precautionary sign to see one's physician. If diagnosed and treated in time by a very wide surgical removal of the involved area, even malignant melanoma can be cured.

So, most skin lesions are benign; those few that are malignant are usually of low grade malignancy. However, since there is the possibility that a rare skin lesion may be of a very serious type, it is always prudent to see your doctor about any new skin growth.

POISON IVY

The most common cause of allergic contact dermatitis in the United States today is that caused by exposure, in sensitive persons, to the toxic products of three plants: poison ivy, poison oak, or poison sumac.

Note the phrase "in sensitive persons" used above, for there is still some medical controversy about just who is susceptible to poison ivy and who is not. (When speaking of *poison ivy* here, one should understand the terms *poison oak* or *poison sumac* also, for there is no way of distinguishing among the rashes caused by any of the three). There are some people who claim they just can't get poison ivy. That statement is still open to debate. What is certainly true is that there are some people who have never *had* poison ivy: But, whether they would not get it after a deliberate exposure to it has never been definitely proved. And there aren't too many volunteers for such a project.

What is certainly agreed upon is that there are an awful lot of people who can get very sick from poison ivy, although there does seem to be some evidence that their reactions tend to diminish as they get older, having experienced intermittent exposure to the weed over the years.

Briefly the poison ivy rash is a cluster of small fluid-filled blisters with some surrounding redness. That is what a typical case looks like. Another clue to its being due to poison ivy is that the rash usually occurs in a linear fashion—that might have resulted from having rubbed up against the plant. A mild case might, however, be manifested just by redness without the blisters, and in a very severe case, the blisters can become quite large.

That's the way it looks. It usually heals in 2 to 3 weeks unless some bacterial infection of the scratched blisters sets in or unless one is reexposed to the offending plant. Unfortunately for all involved, there is no cure. Treatment consists mainly of trying to keep the patient comfortable by relieving the itch until the rash subsides.

In mild-to-moderate poison ivy dermatitis, the main problem is to relieve the itching, because the blisters themselves do not bother the patient too much. The itchiness is best relieved by cool soaks such as dilute Burow's solution which can be purchased from a pharmacy. Tepid cornstarch and baking soda baths are also quite effective in relieving the itchiness. Various shake lotions such as plain calamine lotion are also a good thing to apply directly over the rash to relieve the itching.

Overdrying and cracking of the skin is to be avoided during the acute phase. The application of antihistamines in various forms over the rash has proved to be of no use at all. However, some patients have experienced relief by the use of antihistamines in doses large enough to cause sedation. Others have found that two aspirin every 3 to 4 hours has also produced relief, but this is a lot of aspirin and may lead to gastric irritation. The use of various cortisone compounds, applied either locally to the rash or taken by mouth, can be very helpful but is rarely necessary in mild to moderate poison ivy.

One should also reassure the patient that he cannot give the rash to his family by contact with them. Also the patient should be reassured that he cannot spread it on himself from the blister fluid.

Severe poison ivy is a much more difficult problem because the patient is in great discomfort from the oozing, crusting, itching, and smarting. It is best for such a patient to rest at home using cool compresses for 10 to 15 minutes every 2 to 3 hours. Aspirin and sedatives are useful to relieve the symptoms and to provide the patient with some rest. Cortisone compounds, taken internally, will be very helpful in speeding relief. These latter, however, must be taken only under a doctor's careful supervision because cortisone is a powerful medicine which can have serious side effects.

In order to avoid reexposure to the offending chemical, one should see to it that all possibly contaminated items, such as clothing, sheets, sleeping bags, shoes, etc., should be washed or cleaned. As a matter of fact, the irritating poison ivy oils have been found on such items as rocks, tools, and even automobiles. Such potentially contaminated items should also either be avoided or cleaned. One rare method, luckily, of getting a case of poison ivy in the lungs has been the breathing in of the smoke and fumes from the spring-or-fall cleanup—inadvertent burning of an unrecognized poison ivy vine!

How does one keep from getting this bothersome condition? Barrier creams have not proved too effective. Thorough washing, after exposure, has not prevented the rash in highly sensitive persons, though it may be sufficient for the less sensitive. Some authorities feel that harsh soaps and vigorous scrubbing offer no advantage over simple soaking in cool water.

Finally, there is the possibility of receiving shots to diminish one's sensitivity to poison ivy. These must be done under a doctor's supervision because severe reactions from the shots can, and do, occur. Also the treatment has to be continued from 6 to 12 months a year. It should therefore be reserved for very sensitive persons or for others who, because of their work or environment, just cannot avoid exposure to it.

SUNBURN

A sun tan is one thing. An even-glowing tan looks good and, to a slight extent, even affords a protective shield against sunburn. But that's about its only value. In fact, too much sun exposure ages the skin. It can cause permanent damage and may even lead to skin cancer.

A sunburn is another thing entirely. Too much sun before the skin is tanned means a burn just like the burn produced by fire or a hot iron. With redness, swelling, and pain, blistering, peeling, and itching, it can be sheer misery. You've seen it. You may even have had it. It's no fun, for it can spoil your whole vacation. Here's how to avoid it.

First, some facts about the burning rays of the sun: They are most intense around midday, so, until you're tanned, take your sun in the early morning or late afternoon. The rays penetrate light haze *and* overcast—you don't have to see the sun to get burned. They are reflected by sand and water—you can get burned even while sitting under an umbrella or an awning. Finally, the burning rays are not the heat rays—you can get badly burned on a cool day, especially when it's the breeze that's keeping you from feeling the heat.

The key to avoiding a burn is to take the sun gradually, in installments: a little at first, no more than about 10–15 minutes on each side, then increasing the time as your skin begins to tan. Let your complexion be your guide: light-skinned blondes have to be much more cautious than dark-skinned brunettes.

Persons with a sun allergy have to be especially careful if they want to avoid the itching and hives. Certain drugs and chemicals *(e.g.,* antibiotics, the oil in orange peel, deodorants in some soaps or sprays, etc.) are "sensitizers" that greatly increase susceptibility to sunburn. If you're taking medication, or if you seem to burn too easily, check with your physician.

What about sun creams, lotions, and sprays? Before you buy, decide what you want them to do. Read the labels and, if in doubt, ask the druggist or your doctor.

Most "sun" creams simply contain moisturizers and lubricants to counteract the drying effects of sun, wind, and water. They're soothing, but they do nothing for sunburn.

Some "tanning" creams contain stains or dyes that darken the skin. They're good for "faking" a tan, but don't rely on them for protection, since the burning rays go right through them. The old dodge of putting some iodine in baby oil or mineral oil is in this class—it stains, but it doesn't help the tan or avoid the burn.

Real protection is given by sun-screening preparations (containing para-aminobenzoic acid, salicylates, or benzophenone compounds). A thick coating of zinc oxide ointment will keep all the rays out. The screening creams and lotions do a partial job (depending on how much is applied), allowing you to stay out longer without burning. Remember that they work down into the skin and wash off in the water; be sure to keep reapplying them every hour or two and especially after bathing.

Sunburn preparations can be used if you've been careless. They contain soothing moisturizers and balms often supplemented by benzocaine or some other local anesthetic to stop the pain. (Many people are allergic to these skin anesthetics; they ease the pain temporarily, but make things worse by causing allergic swelling and itching.) Most painful burns respond nicely to cold wet compresses initially and later to cold cream, baby oil, or a soothing lubricant. Severe sunburn with extreme pain or extensive blistering should be treated by your physician to prevent infection and subsequent scarring.

6
Drugs and Medicines

ALCOHOLISM

The following story has been only slightly changed—to protect the guilty:

On a recent rainy morning, a group of us was waiting for an elevator, silently shaking umbrellas or scuffling shoes or nodding in silent sympathy with a neighboring stranger about the downpour. One of us, a middle-aged lady, was really going on in a loud voice. Since her brief remarks did not seem to be evoking any response, I casually looked around to find her probably-embarassed (because her voice was quite loud), soft-spoken friend—only to find no one. That is, she wasn't with anyone nor was she talking to anyone in particular. When one remark bounced off a briefly smiling stranger who then studiously turned away to contemplate his shoes, she turned to someone else with another loud, friendly complaint. Unfortunately, he immediately became occupied with trying to figure out which elevator was going to arrive next.

Eventually, an elevator arrived and we all crowded in. The men who stepped back to let her on first were greeted with such loud friendly disclaimers that they quickly gave up all attempts at courtesy and scuttled as far back in the elevator as possible, in order to contemplate various spots on the walls. By the time I got in, I was standing in front of and slightly to the side of her. The last person on the elevator was a young girl she seemed to know. After a loud greeting, which was answered by a shy smile, our lady continued her comments, in a loud voice, on the state of the world. The young girl looked embarrassed. My stop came and I got off the elevator.

End of story? Not quite. What was really going on in this brief set of encounters which took even less time to happen than it does to relate? Standing as close to her as I was, I think I knew *for sure* what was going on. She reeked of alcohol—a combination of stale and fresh smells on her breath that was no result of a before-or-after dinner drink the evening before. Probably we were dealing with a case of a before-breakfast drink or, more likely, drinks.

The moral of the story is twofold: I'm pretty sure I *knew* what the problem was. I smelled the alcohol, and she was acting as if she was somewhat intoxicated. But I'm sure most of the others didn't *know* what was going on—at least didn't know on a conscious level. But what they did was very interesting. They uniformly avoided her, looked away, were embarrassed; in general, these typical employees ignored her. I'm guessing, however, that, at a subconscious, nonverbal level, they may very well *have* grasped what was going on—but, after all, who wants to get involved in conversation with a drunk?

Unfortunately, it is this very kind of attitude that results in the sweeping under the carpet of problem drinkers as well as their problems. Since the problem is not too common, we can "get away" with our attitude of looking off into space. "After all, nobody's getting hurt." But is that so? Certainly, the drinker's job suffers. His future suffers. His family suffers. His friends suffer. Above all, he suffers. Maybe the more appropriate comment when faced with an alcoholic would be, "After all, who isn't getting hurt?"

So, we learned from Moral Number One that no one individually seems to want to get involved with a drinker. Moral of the Story Number Two is even worse. When I got to my office, I alerted the staff that we would shortly be getting a call from a supervisor about a drunken lady. That call never came! Maybe she's such a top performer that, even under the influence of alcohol, her work doesn't suffer at all—but I doubt it. Maybe she sobered up between the elevator and her desk—but I doubt it. Maybe all traces of alcohol miraculously disappeared from her breath by the time she got to her office—but I doubt it. Maybe her supervisor, acting as an individual, as a "nice guy," looked the other way as everyone else had—I hope not. Maybe he didn't even notice it—then what kind of supervisor is he?

We *are* our brothers' keepers. Alcoholism is a bad thing, whether you belong to the "it's a disease" school, or "it's a moral failing" school, or "it's a character weakness" school. You're not doing him a favor by looking away. By *not* looking away next time, you may help save his job, do his family a real favor, and may help save his life.

To now consider some statistics about alcohol: One highball or cocktail (containing 1-1/2 ounces of whiskey) leads to a blood concentration of alcohol that doesn't leave the body until 2 full hours have gone by. Two drinks require 4 hours to be metabolized; three drinks, 6 hours; and so forth.

Thus five drinks, spaced one every 2 hours for 10 hours, won't make you drunk but will require all that time to be cleared from the blood. Five drinks in a couple of hours will lead to true intoxication with its unmistakable abnormalities of gross bodily functions and mental facilities—and it still requires a full 10 hours before complete clearing of the alcohol from the blood occurs.

This "five drinks in a couple of hours" level is at the 0.15% concentration of alcohol in the blood. At a higher concentration of 0.20%, the drinker is helpless. At 0.30% his brain is almost inoperative, and sensation is so dulled that he no longer sees and hears. At 0.40% to 0.50%, his brain is anesthetized and he is in a coma. At 0.60% his heart stops and so does he.

An interesting series of questions about alcoholism (as contrasted to "social drinking") is worth reviewing to see if one has slipped over into a more serious category altogether.

Does a person

1. Need a drink the "morning after"?
2. Like to drink alone?
3. Lose time from work due to drinking?
4. *Need* a drink at a *definite time* daily?
5. Have a *loss of memory* while or after drinking?
6. Find himself (or others) harder to *get along with?*
7. Find his efficiency and ambition decreasing?
8. Drink to relieve shyness, fear, inadequacy?
9. Find his drinking is *harming* or worrying his family?
10. Find himself more moody, jealous, or irritable after drinking?

If the answers to that list are "yes" (even to just some of the questions), the person is probably suffering from "alcoholism" which is a major problem in itself. It can, however, be arrested if the person recognizes it for what it is.

However, as with all problems, no drinking problem can be solved unless the person with it wants it to be solved. Once he is willing to seek treatment, though, there are a number of resources available to him.

Most large communities either have or are located near a city that has a local chapter of the National Council on Alcoholism. Such agencies are specifically set up to help guide people toward definitive sources of treatment. Moreover, many employers, especially among the larger companies, have established programs in which referral of employees with problems to community resources is a big part.

Before listing some of the various community resources available, I should mention that, to date, there is no acceptable medical evidence that problem drinking is due to some physical or chemical or hormonal imbalance or deficiency of the body. Though in the long run the body is affected, and seriously so, to the point where alcoholism can lead to death, the initiating cause seems to be in the psychological makeup of the person.

What are some of the community treatment resources available to problem drinkers?

1. Alcoholics Anonymous—They have a higher cure rate than any other available approach and the strict confidentiality of their approach, along with their around-the-clock availability, make them an important community resource.
2. One's family doctor—If he has the time for it. If he doesn't, he may be able to recommend others who do.
3. A psychiatrist—Preferably one who has worked with such problems before.
4. One's minister, rabbi, or priest.
5. An alcoholism clinic in a nearby hospital.
6. Short-term hospitalization in special clinics.
7. Selected psychologists or social workers who have had experience with such problems.

These are some of the resources available if only the patient will take advantage of them.

ASPIRIN

Aspirin is still one of the best of all medications available to doctors—yet, how many people take it for granted or, even worse, assume that their doctor has tried to "put something over" on them because "all he prescribed was aspirin."

From ancient times it was known that various extracts of the bark of the willow tree were effective in lowering elevated body temperatures, but it wasn't until the 1830's that the active ingredients in that bark were identified. This set of chemicals is called the salicylates from the Latin name for willow tree: *Salix.* By far the most widely used of all the salicylates is acetylsalicylic acid, or aspirin, as it is more commonly called.

Like most medicines that are at all effective, aspirin has side effects, ranging from the merely unpleasant to the serious.

The most important of all the side effects is the very irritating effect that aspirin (even aspirin combined with a buffering agent) can have on the lining of the stomach. Not only can it cause stomach ache, nausea, and vomiting, but it can actually cause bleeding from the stomach. Now in normal people this bleeding is usually in very small amounts (but it is not unknown to cause anemia over a long period of chronic administration); however, in people with irritable stomachs or ulcers, the blood loss can at times be significant and dangerous. How can one circumvent such a side effect? Take aspirin with or after food, or with milk. Take a form that dissolves rapidly so that its irritant effect is dispersed and diluted rapidly.

Mild rashes can occur in persons who are allergic to aspirin. In very high, really in massive, doses, aspirin can cause ringing in the ears—but this is an uncommon side effect that responds immediately to diminution of the dose.

What about the widely-held belief that too much aspirin can affect the heart? Well, that widely-held belief is widely not held by doctors. In its usual dose, aspirin has no adverse effect on the heart. (As a matter of fact, it helps the heart afflicted by rheumatic fever.)

Aspirin in high doses has some complex effects on metabolism which, while insignificant in adults, can make a child seriously ill, which is one very good reason why aspirin as well as other medications should be kept out of the reach of children. Finally, too high a dosage can actually cause aspirin poisoning which can, in severe cases, result in death. All of this should indicate that aspirin is not a drug that should be taken lightly or for no good reason; unfortunately, it is used indiscriminately by many people for every conceivable ailment.

One of the most important of all the things that aspirin *does* do is to lower fever. It should not, however, be taken just because a person has an elevated temperature. It is probably true that fevers are the body's way of reacting to an illness and that the actual fever may help get rid of that illness. But, when the fever is so high that it is potentially dangerous to the patient (such as, in certain children, high enough to cause convulsions) or when the patient is very uncomfortable and restless because of the fever, then aspirin really comes into its own as perhaps *the* single best drug known for this purpose. We're not too sure of how aspirin achieves many of its effects, but it is believed that part of temperature lowering follows from the sweating that aspirin causes. In a person who has become so dehydrated from the fever that he can't sweat, not only will aspirin not work but it may actually *raise* his temperature. So, when using it in the face of elevated temperatures, make sure the person is also taking lots of fluids.

The next great category of aspirin effectiveness is in the relief of pain. It works for almost all types of pain from headaches and muscular aches through dysmenorrhea, neuralgia, and even arthritis. Again, we don't know how it works: It may actually be dulling the sensation of pain in the brain. There is some evidence, however, that it actually helps relieve the inflammation in the involved part. Very important in this respect is that chronic use does not lead to tolerance (requiring higher and higher doses) nor to addiction (with its physical-psychological dependence on the drug).

A corollary to the possible dulling effect on the brain's pain awareness is another effect for which aspirin is used: as a tranquilizer. Aspirin does seem to cause brain wave changes similar to those caused by some tranquilizers, which may explain what's going on in those many people who take "a couple of aspirin" to help them get to sleep.

One use of aspirin which is questionable is, unfortunately, one of the most common: its use in "colds" and other minor respiratory infections. Aspirin does *nothing* to prevent or cure or shorten the course of a cold. Sure, it will relieve the fever and the muscular aching that go with a cold, but there is some real evidence that a cold may last longer if you load up with aspirin than if you just let it run its course. Incidentally, for all the good that a gargle containing aspirin does, you might just as well use it as a hair rinse.

One of the most dramatic of the uses of aspirin is in acute rheumatic fever. Again, we don't know how it works, but usually the affected person will experience, within 24–48 hours after adequate doses of aspirin, considerable or complete relief of pain, swelling, immobility, and the heat and redness of the involved joints. The fever and the pulse rate are lowered, and the patient usually feels much better. While aspirin does not really shorten the course of the disease, nor does it really control the disease, it certainly helps lessen the severity of its manifestations and often can abort the secondary complications that would have followed the completely unchecked expression of the rheumatic fever.

Aspirin is the mainstay of treatment in that crippling form of arthritis known as rheumatoid arthritis. It relieves pain and increases appetite and a feeling of well-being. Besides these nonspecific effects, aspirin definitely reduces the inflammation of the joints and the surrounding tissues. As a result it lessens or, at least, delays the development of crippling. One would have to reach into the cortisone category of drugs to find some medicine as effective.

It is because of its "joint-sparing" effect as well as its pain relief that aspirin is also widely used for the noncrippling form of arthritis, called osteoarthritis.

One relatively rare use of aspirin in high doses is to increase the urinary excretion of uric acid, thus diminishing the possibility of stone formation in patients with gout.

Finally, a new use for aspirin has recently been reported. Though much more research is required before it achieves a permanent place on the therapeutic shelf, aspirin seems also to be effective in preventing heart attacks. As might have been predicted, once again we do not know how aspirin exerts this prophylactic effect, but one theory is that it serves as a sort of blood-thinner since it *is* known that aspirin can cause a bleeding tendency in some people and does prolong the time it takes for blood to clot. This may be secondary to a diminution of the stickiness of the blood platelets (which are a factor in blood clotting).

The uses of aspirin do not end here, but the other conditions are rarer and the proof that aspirin has much of an effect in them is shakier.

DRIVING AND DRINKING

Bad habits are bad enough. When they can kill us they're even worse; but when our bad habits kill other people, then things really are in terrible shape. I suspect that the majority of Americans do believe that cigarette smoking is a bad habit; and that in the right person (or, rather, in the *wrong* person), it can actually indirectly shorten the life span or can even be the direct cause of death such as via lung cancer. But in the long run, the cigarette smoker's bad habit is only going to hurt *him* directly.

A bad habit that *can* kill others is driving when drinking. We're not saying that all drinking is bad, but we are saying that all driving after drinking is bad. Maybe it's not a habit; maybe it's just carelessness—but, however one labels it, an awful lot of Americans do drive after drinking and, as a result, are killing themselves—and others.

Recent statistics which have been released in Washington by the Secretary of Transportation are frightening. "The use of alcohol by drivers and pedestrians leads to some 25,000 deaths and a total of at least 800,000 crashes in the United States each year." Those figures are of epidemic proportions, but Americans seem to greet them with a sort of "it can't happen to me" indifference. If influenza, for example, killed 25,000 people a year, we'd probably be in a state of panic trying to control the epidemic. As a matter of fact, even though influenza as a killer is not anywhere near the same league, millions of Americans get their flu shots each year in their attempt to do something about it.

The problem then is: How do we get Americans to do something about this epidemic of manslaughter on the American highways? Maybe we can let the facts speak for themselves.

Repeated investigations have shown that immoderate use of alcohol is a very major source of highway crashes and that it contributes to about half of all highway deaths. There is another aspect of the problem that is even more discouraging. Recent research has shown that more than half of adults in America use the highways at least occasionally after drinking!

The real killers, however, seem to be men who have been drinking heavily. Thus, while problem drinkers constitute only a small proportion of the population, they account for a very large part of the overall problem.

The tragedy of the situation is that the drinking driver not only kills himself but often kills nondrinking, innocent persons that he happens to run into. When is this most likely to happen? Again, the Secretary of Transportation's report indicates that while crashes involving alcohol occur at all times of the day, they are relatively uncommon during morning rush hours. The majority of alcohol-involved crashes occur during the late afternoon, evening, and night-time hours. The other side of the coin is also true: Most of the late-in-the-day traffic crashes will be found to have alcohol as a significant contributing factor. In one study the odds were more than eight to one that the driver fatally injured in a single vehicle crash between 9 P.M. and midnight had been drinking heavily.

These evening alcohol-related crashes are common on all days of the week because heavy drinkers generally do not confine their abuse of alcohol to weekends, but such accidents are especially common on Saturdays when the non-problem-drinker, social drinkers, are added to that pool of irresponsible Americans who drive after drinking.

The figures should speak for themselves. They are horrible—and our national indifference is also terrible. And yet what will you do about it? Would you consider *walking* to that New Year's Eve party? Or using public transportation only? Or, funnier still, would you consider driving to that New Year's Eve party and then not taking a drink? Would you rather kill somebody because you drove while drinking, or would you just rather be killed by someone who drove while drinking?

DRUGS AND DRIVING

A reminder to physicians about drugs and driving appeared in a leading medical journal. Since even physicians tend to forget the importance of the relationship between drugs and automobile accidents, it might be valuable to reemphasize some of these really frightening facts for the layman, who may also have let them slip from his mind or, worse still, who may not originally have been warned about them by his doctor.

We all know how important alcohol is as a cause of traffic accidents and fatalities, but we may not be aware that alcohol is, technically speaking, just one of a larger category of compounds–drugs in general. Because the current estimate is that over 50% of highway accidents occur because of the ingestion of alcohol (not necessarily always to the level of "intoxication") on the part of one or both involved parties, the emphasis has rightly been placed on the "if you're going to drive, don't drink" approach.

What is generally *not* realized, however, is that a significant percentage of the remaining traffic accidents involve persons under the influence of "drugs"–and we don't mean just "junkies" or "wild kids on LSD." The growing problem in traffic is concerned with a host of medicines legitimately used and prescribed, often taken indiscriminately, and *always potentially dangerous.*

The chief "nonalcohol" offending drugs that are being implicated in driving accidents include the more obvious true narcotics such as heroin, morphine, demerol, and codeine, as well as the less obvious categories of sedatives such as phenobarbital, tranquilizers such as Miltown and Librium, and (the real "sleepers") antihistamines such as just about everybody seems to be taking most of the time for myriad reasons (especially since these drugs are contained in most motion sickness, allergy, and cold remedies). These and other drugs acting on the central nervous system can adversely affect alertness, motor coordination, skills, judgment, and other faculties essential for safe driving.

Perhaps the most important fact leading to the general lack of awareness regarding the effects of nonalcoholic drugs on driving is that only a very small amount of them is required to cause a pronounced effect, whereas some several ounces of alcohol are needed to yield a comparable intoxication. When it is recalled that even low levels of alcohol (certainly short of "intoxication") lead to impairment of driving skills, then the importance of drug effects falls into more proper perspective. Also to be emphasized is the fact that even small drug quantities are only slowly destroyed or metabolized in the human body, so that rather extended effects result from even low doses, while alcohol is generally destroyed at the rate of 1/3 to 1/2 ounce per hour!

Thus, a medical article, in commenting on one of the most widely used of the tranquilizers, noted that even though the manufacturer's recommended dose is 15 to 100 mg daily, the ingestion of just 20 mg a day for 1 week had the following results: "judgment scores were poorer" and "subjects were more likely to increase their speed with a concomitant decrease in accuracy."

Even the stimulants such as amphetamine "pep pills" paradoxically diminish rather than increase one's efficiency; their euphoric effects have been shown to impair judgment and have resulted in drivers taking excessive risks.

Very recently it has been reported that one of the less commonly used antibiotics, Negram, has on occasion been responsible for "drowsiness, fatigue and reversible subjective visual disturbances such as overbrightness of lights, change in visual color perception, difficulty in focusing, decrease in visual acuity and double vision."

Most serious of all is the combination of alcohol with any of the above preparations. This drug-alcohol combination in many instances can produce a synergistic or mutual-aid effect whereby each enhances the effect of the other, so that 1 plus 1 may no longer make 2 but may result in 4 or 5 units of effect.

What then is to be done about all this? Obviously, drug manufacturers should advise physicians of any "driving side-effects" of their drugs. Well, in most cases they do. What then? Physicians should then pass on the warnings to their patients. Such follow-through is, unfortunately, far from 100%. But there's nothing to keep patients from asking their doctors a simple life-saving question such as, "Will this drug impair my driving ability in any way?"

Basically, however, the solution lies in the less-indiscriminate prescription of such drugs by physicians and the avoidance of driving under their influence by patients who *have* to take them.

TOXIC SOLVENTS

In spite of proper labeling of containers and in spite of general public knowledge of their danger, chemical solvents still account each year for a significant number of illnesses and even death. When you add to this the untold number of headaches, dizziness, or eye irritation that occur while painting or cleaning furniture or otherwise using these various chemical solvents, the problem indeed becomes a real one.

Among the most commonly used solvents are carbon tetrachloride, acetone, benzene, turpentine, and wood alcohol. Perhaps the most widely used is carbon tetrachloride whose sweetish odor is easily recognized by most people, many of whom do not consider it particularly disagreeable. Since carbon tetrachloride is both very penetrating and quick drying, it is used in most cleaning fluids. Since it is also fireproof, it is used as the basic fluid in many fire extinguishers and extensively used as a basis for oils, grease, paints, waxes, and rubber compounds. It is also used as a fumigating mixture and can be used as an insecticide. Carbon tetrachloride is a highly toxic material. Acute exposure can cause irritation of the upper respiratory tract, as well as injury to the lungs, liver, and kidneys; the latter can be and, unfortunately, too often is fatal. It also causes tearing of the eyes even at low levels of exposure.

(In recognition of the extreme toxicity of carbon tetrachloride, the Food and Drug Administration has banned its use in products, including fire extinguishers, intended for *household* and *residential* use, effective November 19, 1970. It was impossible to write precautionary labeling sufficient to protect the public.)

Acetone is another quick-drying (which really means highly-vaporizable) solvent used in varnishes, lacquers, plastics, and rubber production, but more importantly for our purposes as a solvent for removing stains in clothing and in many glues. It is its use in the latter that accounted for the outbreak of "glue sniffing" that has been making the scene in the past few years. As, hopefully, everyone knows by now, such "trips" have led to blindness and even death. Routine exposure, however, though not so dangerous, can cause eye irritation and nose and throat irritation.

Benzene is a common basis for some rubber and plastic cements. It is also found in paints, varnish removers, quick-drying inks, and insecticides. Among the side effects of high benzene vapor exposure are, first, a feeling of exhilaration followed by drowsiness, fatigue, vertigo, nausea, and headache. With even higher concentrations or longer exposures, convulsion, paralysis, and unconsciousness may occur. Even death has occurred following an acute exposure. Chronic exposure to repeated small amounts of benzene vapor is of greater importance, for this can cause various blood abnormalities such as low red blood cell count, low white blood cell count, and even fatal bone marrow damage.

Finally, turpentine and wood alcohol are known as thinners for paints, varnishes, and lacquers and are generally used for cleaning brushes, hardware, and hands after painting. Turpentine can cause irritation of the mucous membranes of the eyes and nose with acute exposure. Headache, dizziness, nausea, chest pain, and sometimes visual disturbances have been reported following high concentration exposure. Even transient kidney damage has been reported following such exposure.

Unfortunately, methyl alcohol does not have a suitable warning odor or mucous membrane irritating properties except at high concentrations. It is, however, potentially, one of the most dangerous of solvents, for the list of its complications after high dose vapor inhalation is long indeed: irritation of all the mucous membranes, headache, roaring in the ears, tiredness, insomnia, trembling, dizziness, unsteady gait, shortness of breath, nausea, vomiting, colic, dilated pupils, clouded vision, double vision, and, worst of all, blindness.

With such prevalent and dangerous side effects, it logically follows that no solvents should be used in closed or poorly ventilated spaces. Ideally, adequate ventilation means working outdoors. If that is impractical, then doors and windows should be opened. If possible, a low-placed fan should be used to exhaust the fumes. Of course, none of those solvents should be stored in an open container because they are all highly vaporizable and it is their vapors that can cause the damage.

Each of these compounds is extremely toxic if ingested, with even relatively small amounts (on the order of one teaspoonful) causing the most serious side effects including, in the case of some of them, blindness and death.

So, when handling solvents follow carefully all the recommendations on the labels of the containers. The use of protective gloves is a good idea. If there is any skin contact, the skin should be immediately washed thoroughly with soap and water for absorption can occur through the unbroken skin. Clothing that may have absorbed fumes should be given a chance to "air out." And certainly all such solvents should be kept out of the reach of children.

If overexposure has occurred, it is imperative to remove the victim from the possibility of further contact with the chemical. Mouth-to-mouth resuscitation may be required if breathing has stopped. Aside from these two emergency first aid measures, treatment of solvent intoxication should be guided by a physician.

With proper precautions, some of these solvents such as turpentine and acetone can be used in the home without ill effect. But remember, solvent intoxication deserves as much caution as cancer or heart disease—since it can be just as fatal!

7
Eyes

COMMON EYE DISORDERS

About 8 years ago The Food and Drug Administration announced steps to make safety glasses mandatory in virtually all the new eyeglasses Americans wear. This was an excellent proposal for it has been estimated that 120,000 persons are injured each year by accidents in which the eyeglass lenses are shattered.

An even more startling statistic is that 100 million Americans (just a little less than half of all Americans) wear prescription eyeglasses. What are all these people wearing all those glasses for? They do so either because of farsightedness, nearsightedness, or astigmatism.

Briefly, the eyeball is a spherical container with the pupillary opening in the front to let the light rays in, a form of crystalline lens almost directly behind it to help focus the incoming rays of light, and a light-sensing area called the retina lining the back of the sphere.

Generally there are few, if any, problems that arise because of pupillary malfunction. Normally the pupil dilates in the dark (to let in more light) or when it is focusing on something in the distance, and it constricts in bright light or for close visual work. Just as rare as pupillary causes of visual difficulties in eyeglass wearers are retinal problems. The retina lies over the inner surface of the sphere, and unless it detaches (in which case actual blindness can result) or has some congenital abnormality of its structure, it usually functions without problems.

We are left then with abnormal lens curvatures or cloudings as one cause of visual difficulties. Thus, on occasion diabetics will notice a sudden onset or worsening of nearsightedness. This is probably due to an increase, in diabetics, of the fluid content of the lens which in turn increases its curvature. Cataracts are a form of clouding of the lens that usually occurs in older persons, and this clouding also would obviously lead to loss of clarity of vision as well as to some alterations in the normal paths of the light waves.

But even lens abnormalities are not the most common cause of visual problems that lead to the wearing of eyeglasses. The most common cause of these refractive errors is an abnormality in the shape of the sphere itself.

Hyperopia or farsightedness, which is the most common of the refractive errors, is due in most cases to such an abnormal shape of the eyeball. In such cases the eyeball is too short from front to back. As a result the rays of light actually would come to a focus in back of the retina. The principal cause of this, as well as of all the other errors of refraction, is heredity. Of course there is one type of farsightedness which is not hereditary: When the entire lens of the eye is removed because of cataracts (or cloudings) of the lens, the eye becomes very far-sighted indeed.

Farsighted persons notice no problem when viewing objects at a distance. It's when objects are close at hand (such as reading) that they experience difficulty. Such persons may complain of pain in the eye after prolonged use, blurring of the print while reading, and even on occasion may experience headaches. When these symptoms are severe and not corrected by glasses, reading may become impossible. Some eye doctors feel that it is really a basic, severe, inherited farsightedness that is responsible for some of the "cross eyed" conditions seen in young children.

A visit to an eye *doctor* should precede the obtaining of corrective lenses for farsightedness. If the condition is only a mild one, eyeglasses may not be required, especially if the patient is not experiencing any symptoms. When glasses are prescribed, they are usually needed, at first, for reading and close work only. As the person gets older, he may eventually have to wear them not only for reading but all the time. Actually there can be added to this basic farsightedness changes due to aging, so that by the time such a person gets to be 45 or 50 years of age, he will have to have either two pairs of glasses—

one for reading and one for distance—or he will require bifocals with the upper part of the lens ground to a distance correction and the lower part ground to a reading correction.

Nearsightedness or myopia occurs in the eyeball that is too long. In such an eye the image comes to a focus in front of the retina, and what actually gets to the retina is a blurred image. Again, as in farsightedness, the most important cause is heredity—a hereditary asymmetry of eyeball growth. This is why most nearsighted persons become symptomatic during adolescence and young adulthood. Once growth is complete, the nearsighted eye usually stabilizes and does not continue to get worse. The controversy as to whether close work (such as school work or reading) in youthful years causes myopia is still unresolved, but most eye doctors now are generally agreed that there is no good evidence that the use of the eyes in any way changes the degree of myopia or is, in any way, detrimental to eyes having an ordinary degree of myopia. Myopes usually have no symptoms other than an awareness that they cannot see at a distance so well as other persons.

The treatment of nearsightedness is corrective lenses prescribed by an eye *doctor.* Some eye doctors believe that if myopes wear their glasses faithfully and regularly, they will prevent any progressive worsening of their vision. Unfortunately there is no real evidence to support this. As far as eye exercises for nearsightedness go, again there is no proof that they have any effect on the condition, although they are probably not harmful.

An interesting occurrence sometimes is present in myopes who are not too severe to begin with. As they get older, they begin, in their 30's and 40's to get the to-be-expected changes of presbyopia (farsightedness which occurs in the older person). As a result they often find that they will require a weakening of their eyeglass prescription, and some rare cases have even found that they no longer needed eyeglasses because, for a while at least, their presbyopia exactly counterbalanced their myopia. However, presbyopia, though not so rapidly progressing as myopia, nonetheless continues, and eventually even these patients will probably need glasses for near vision.

One complication seen more often in the nearsighted rather than the farsighted eye is detachment of the retina. It's as if the long eyeball is actually being placed under a stretch form of tension which can ultimately (though, luckily, rarely) result in actual retinal detachment. That's why those with a high degree of myopia are often cautioned against such violent sports as boxing, football, or high diving.

Astigmatism is the third chief cause of errors of refraction. In this case it is the cornea or outer shell in front of the eye that is at fault. Where normally the cornea has a spherical curvature like the inside of a kitchen bowl, in astigmatism the corneal curvature is like that of a kitchen spoon.

Again the cause is heredity. The symptoms that result may be headache and pain after using the eyes, especially after activity requiring prolonged attention at a distance, such as attending the theater or driving. And, of course, the vision is blurred. The treatment is the wearing of corrective lenses at all times.

A final word as to the type of specialists who work with eye patients. An ophthalmologist is the same thing as an oculist. Both are M.D.'s who, after completing their basic training, went on and specialized in eye diseases. They often are the physicians who give patients prescriptions for corrective glasses. They are not, however, those who fill the prescriptions. The optometrist is in the middle ground, so to speak, between an ophthalmologist and an optician. An optometrist has the right training to prescribe corrective lenses and often has the facilities to fill those prescriptions. Unlike an ophthalmologist, however, he is not competent to diagnose and treat complex eye diseases nor to do eye surgery. Finally, an optician is an eyeglass specialists, so to speak. Opticians do not write prescriptions for lenses; rather they fit the patient with the right frame and the right lenses from prescriptions of either an ophthalmologist or optometrist.

Many patients have mentioned to me that their ophthalmologist, being so highly specialized in some of the very complex aspects of eye surgery and diseases, was less willing to spend a lot of time in writing a prescription for new eyeglasses for them than they found when they had visited optometrists, and this may very well be the case. This is not to deny that ophthalmologists are happy to write prescriptions, but this is to state that in this area at least a good optometrist is often equal to a good ophthalmologist.

A word of advice. If you are really dependent on your eyeglasses to keep you from joining the ranks of the walking wounded, keep a second pair handy for emergencies.

GLAUCOMA

Thanks to the efficiency of mass media communications, when one says "glaucoma" to someone, quite often they will remember the well-advertised slogan, "the sneak thief of sight." If you ask them what *that* means, you just as often run into a blank expression; for while millions may recognize the name "glaucoma," few really know what the disease is all about.

The eyeball can be considered to be a closed spherical object. There is a very thin membrane, the conjunctiva, covering the external part of the eye. Directly behind it is the thicker protective layer called the cornea. Behind that is the anterior chamber of the eye which is divided from the much smaller posterior chamber by the colored iris (this is what gives our eyes their brown or blue color). The iris has a central opening, called the pupil, which can enlarge and constrict, thereby governing the amount of light that enters the eye through the crystalline lens which is at the back of the posterior chamber. There's a lot more of critical importance behind that lens, but the above anatomy is all we need to know to get some idea of what glaucoma is about.

There is a constant internal pressure inside the eyeball of 25 mm mercury or less. One of the chief determinants of that pressure is that amount of aqueous humor present at any one moment in the eye. This liquid, which bathes the structures in front of the lens (the anterior and posterior chambers and the iris), is constantly being formed and eliminated. The rates of production and absorption are so delicately balanced that under normal conditions the intraocular pressure is kept at a relatively constant level. Anything which upsets this level, such as an increase or decrease in either formation or absorption, will result in a change in intraocular pressure unless both processes undergo an equal and simultaneous change.

What then is glaucoma? It's a disease caused by increased intraocular tension which can lead to impairment of vision ranging from slight abnormalities to absolute blindness. There are two main forms of glaucoma: primary and secondary.

The causes of primary glaucoma are unknown. Heredity and farsightedness are for sure among the predisposing factors. Less sure but nonetheless so considered by some are emotional and/or vascular instability. The increase in intraocular tension is caused by an obstruction to the *outflow* of intraocular fluid. Primary glaucoma is of two forms: wide angle, open, chronic simple glaucoma which is caused by actual obstruction of the fluid-exit pores; and narrow angle, acute congestive glaucoma in which there is a shallow anterior chamber making for a narrowing of the filtration angle. A dilated pupil may actually push the root of the iris forward against the angle and can thus precipitate an acute attack. Incidentally, glaucoma is not caused or made worse by using the eyes, and is not due to high blood pressure.

The wide angle, open, chronic simple glaucoma is the most common form. It is characterized by a slow insidious course, with progressive loss of peripheral vision, followed later by loss of central vision. This form is usually bilateral. It should be suspected in any patient, especially if over age 40, who requires frequent changes of lenses, has mild headaches or vague visual disturbances, sees halos around electric lights, or has impaired adaptation of his vision in the dark. The diagnosis is made by tonometry which is the application of a pressure-measuring instrument to the eyeball. Every eye examination of those near or past 40 should include tonometry. The treatment of simple glaucoma involves eyedrops which constrict the pupils, the avoidance of fatigue, emotional upsets, tobacco, and large quantities of fluids. If these don't work, then surgery to increase the filtration is required.

Narrow angle acute congestive glaucoma often may have transitory attacks of diminished vision, colored haloes around lights, and some pain in the eye and head. These attacks may last only a few hours and recur at intervals of weeks to years before a typical prolonged attack of acute glaucoma occurs. The acute attack is characterized by rapid loss of sight and sudden onset of severe throbbing pain in the eye. Nausea and vomiting are frequent. There is considerable swelling of the lids, tearing, and redness of the conjunctiva. The internal eye pressure is considerably increased. With each recurrent attack, vision becomes progressively poorer. Although the usual acute attack is confined to one eye, the other eye is not immune to subsequent acute attacks. The treatment of acute glaucoma involves the systemic use of dehydrators. Pupillary constrictors are also indicated. Surgery can prevent further attacks.

There is a form known as *chronic* narrow angle glaucoma in which the symptoms and signs resemble those of acute glaucoma, but all are less severe than in the acute form.

Secondary glaucoma is caused by any blockage of aqueous humor flow from the posterior chamber through the pupil into the anterior chamber and from there to the exit canals. Internal eye inflammations, eye injuries with subsequent internal scars, intraocular tumors, enlarged cataracts—all have been implicated. In this form, in addition to the treatments listed above, the use of cortisone compounds may be helpful.

Once the diagnosis is made, it is advisable to visit an ophthalmologist at regular intervals for the rest of one's life because glaucoma can, indeed, be "the sneak thief of sight."

8
Gastrointestinal

APPENDICITIS

In the past 10 to 20 years, one has heard rather less of appendicitis than one used to, and the reasons for this are not at all too clear. Whether there has been a real lessening of the frequency of appendicitis as some doctors claim, or whether diagnostic accuracy has increased to the point where more accurate other diagnoses are being made so that fewer normal appendices are being removed, or whether the use of antibiotics has contributed to this lessening is unclear. It may even be an artificial slipping out of current awareness due to the relatively easy nature and almost routine aspect of appendectomies.

One interesting thing that has been learned about the appendix in general is that it is not quite the useless internal organ that it was once believed to be. It turns out that the appendix is part of the body's lymphoid defensive system. In some lower animals, it is a relatively large appendage to the junction of the small intestine with the large intestine and serves as a source of lymphocytes (or white blood cells) which makes those blood chemicals that help prevent and control infections. Certainly, it is true that in humans the appendix is relatively smaller than it is in these other animals. The human body also contains, scattered along the lower part of the small intestine, patches of lymph tissue which serve as its chemical defense function. It is as if this function in man is diffused; but the appendix still retains an important part of it. In short, as I have said before, whoever put the body together may well have known what he was doing: The appendix is not useless. Some statistics a few years ago showed that the frequency of cancer of the large intestine (which can be considered downstream from the scavenging function of the appendix) is considerably higher in persons who have had their appendix removed than in those who still retain it.

This is not to say that the appendix should never be removed. Many a person has died because a diagnosis of appendicitis was not made in time, and the condition progressed to perforation, perhaps even widespread peritonitis and abscesses. Before the advent of antibiotics, these latter conditions were very frequently fatal; and even nowadays with antibiotics their treatment is still quite complex, making these conditions something one wishes to avoid at almost all costs. In an attempt to prevent the still dreaded complications of a neglected appendix, the old surgical maxim is still true that a good surgeon will often have to remove, in his career, perfectly normal appendices as an indication that his index of suspicion was high enough.

The appendix is like an earthworm, being anywhere from 2 to 6 inches long, and in its uninflamed state not much thicker than a lead pencil. The reason that it so often causes a problem is that it has a relatively narrow opening leading into it. If a particle of undigested food or a small seed from a fruit, for example, should get into the very narrow canal of the appendix, there may be enough subsequent inflammation around it that the opening becomes so swollen that the particle cannot be expelled. The appendix becomes further engorged by the subsequent inflammation and soon becomes infected, because that part of the large intestine is literally loaded with bacteria, the great majority of which are helpful to the body in digesting and absorbing food and even in helping make necessary food nutrients. Some of these bacteria, however, can become virulent.

An interesting fact about appendicitis is that there is some strong evidence that it may be hereditary. How, one may ask, can an infection be hereditary, because, after all, appendicitis is basically an infection. It is really like an internal boil. How that be hereditary? What is hereditary is the length and shape and sometimes even the position of the appendix. People who inherit long, twisted appendices, which actually are twisted towards the back and upward, seem to run higher risks of having something get stuck in them than persons who have shorter and straighter appendices.

The first symptom of appendicitis is usually pain around the navel. Everyone thinks the pain is in the lower right side of the abdomen, and in most cases it does shift there after the first 3 to 6 hours, but in almost all cases the discomfort and pain begin around the navel. Shortly thereafter there is a feeling of lack of appetite which generally progresses to true nausea and vomiting.

Frequently upon questioning, the person with an attack of appendicitis will describe an unusual presence of a few days constipation; this, in a person who usually doesn't have constipation. Yet one cannot rely on constipation absolutely preceding appendicitis because 10% have diarrhea beforehand. Within about 3 to 6 hours, the pain does shift down to the right side and tends to become continuous. The pain may be either dull or severe, coughing or sneezing can aggravate it, and there is definite tenderness in the area. Almost invariably there is a low-grade fever of up to about 102 degrees. It is most unusual for an uncomplicated attack of acute appendicitis to run a fever higher than 102. This fever, however, is not an early sign. Another finding that the attack can elicit after blood testing is a high white blood cell count.

The taking of laxatives in the presence of symptoms as described above is definitely a bad idea. For one thing, laxatives tend to increase the propulsive and expulsive movements of the intestine. Now, with an acute appendicitis, you have a blocked little organ that is trying to squeeze out a trapped piece of its contents, and it has not succeeded in getting it out through the opening. Taking a laxative increases the squeezing motions of the entire gastrointestinal tract. They can become even more vigorous in the appendix, still unsuccessfully, however. The pressure then rises higher and higher until an actual blowout (perforation) of the appendix can occur. If there ever was a time when a person should be brought to have a physician examine him, it is when one suspects the presence of acute appendicitis.

CIRRHOSIS

One common misconception among many "popular ideas" about medicine is that cirrhosis of the liver is exclusively the result of chronic alcoholism. Doctors have long known that this is not so.

What is cirrhosis of the liver? It's a chronic disease whose underlying mechanism is a serious distortion of the normal structural architecture of the liver. If we cut out skin deeply enough, we get a subsequent scar which will always remain visible as different from the nearby surrounding skin. If a person has a coronary and recovers, the involved portion of his heart will always show the distortion from normal structural appearance due to the thick scar which results as the damaged heart heals.

And so it is with the liver. Cirrhosis can be viewed as the serious widespread scarring of the liver that results *whenever* the liver is subject to serious damage. While it is true that alcoholism is *one* of the causes of cirrhosis, it is not the only cause. Alcohol damages the liver in at least two ways:

1. The alcoholic tends to slip into a chronic habit of eating poorly or not at all. This results in significant changes in liver metabolism and function due to such factors as vitamin deficiencies and lack of proteins. Such changes in metabolism can become progressively more severe so that finally actual structural liver damage can occur. Then the scarring sets in and cirrhosis follows.

2. Alcohol has recently been shown to have a direct toxic or poisonous effect on the liver cells themselves. This may seem obvious to those who do know that alcoholism is *one* of the causes of cirrhosis, but for a number of years doctors believed that such an "obvious" explanation was not an actual fact and that the sole reason for liver damage in alcoholics was due to the dietary malnutrition changes just outlined. The very latest studies, however, have finally confirmed that, besides the malnutrition that accompanies alcoholism, alcohol does have a direct effect on liver cells so that it actually poisons their metabolism and can cause cell death. Thus the cycle is started: Cell damage leads to cell death which leads to scarring which leads to cirrhosis.

Another very frequent cause of cirrhosis is hepatitis. Hepatitis is a relatively common infectious disease of the liver. Luckily for most patients, after a few weeks of jaundice and poor appetite, they get better and that's the end of it. Some people, however, get over the illness on the surface, but there is enough smoldering damage that continues for years or enough initial damage from the primary illness that serious scarring results. Unfortunately, there is no way of telling which persons who've had hepatitis in the past have this scarring going on unless one actually does a biopsy of the liver (which means putting a needle into the liver and taking out a small piece). This is not an innocuous procedure and would mean subjecting a lot of people to it—which really wouldn't be worth it from an overall point of view for two reasons: (1) It's definitely a minority of persons who have had hepatitis who then go on to develop cirrhosis, and (2) even if one could detect the scarring process in that minority there is at present no practical medical means to prevent its progression.

Another cause of cirrhosis (in this case it is called biliary cirrhosis) is chronic blocking of the flow of bile from the liver, such as from an impacted gallstone, or scarring around the gallbladder from previous surgery, or some congenital narrowing of the passages down which bile flows from the liver to the gallbladder and eventually to the intestines. This form of cirrhosis of quite rare.

Still another cause of cirrhosis, though an uncommon one, is chronic heart failure which leads to almost constant liver congestion and swelling and which can lead, in some cases, to liver cell damage and then scarring.

Very rare causes of cirrhosis are certain diseases of metabolism such as Wilson's desease which is due to an abnormal accumulation of copper in the liver, which causes cell damage. This is a congenital defect as may be hemochromatosis which is due to an abnormal deposition of iron in the liver (although there are some cases where it seems that hemochromatosis is not due to a congenital defect but rather to an excess ingestion of medicinal iron for prolonged periods of time).

Finally there is idiopathic cirrhosis. Idiopathic is a fancy word for "we don't know," but in these cases all the above causes have been pretty well ruled out.

CONSTIPATION

How often are we regaled in our T.V. commericals or other media with the image and voice of a kindly, white-haired motherly figure with a look of concern on her face, a knowing look in her eye, and words of wisdom to one and all about what to do for their constipation.

In this pill-oriented culture of ours, there are many patent medications for those worried Americans who enjoy contemplating their bowels. The detrimental result has been not only a burgeoning of liquids and pills, suppositories, and enemas on your friendly druggist's counter, but even more unfortunate has been the promulgation of a philosophy of health among Americans that espouses a daily bowel movement as being normal. Many an American hastens to the medicine cabinet in concern over the psychological discomfort of having missed his daily b.m.

There are in fact very rare occasions when medical practice would warrant the use of a laxative (or cathartic as the grey-haired mother would speak of it). If someone has ingested a dangerous drug or some form of toxic food (either one of which can result in poisoning), a saline laxative is often recommended to help rid the intestinal tract of the offending agent. People who are afflicted with various worms in the intestinal tract are often told to take a laxative along with their "deworming" pills. People who are going to have X-rays of their intestine or stomach are often told to take a laxative prior to their examination. A laxative or an enema is often used prior to a proctoscopic examination.

Having listed the above, all of which, obviously, are relatively rare but, nonetheless, valid indications for the use of laxatives or enemas, we find much to the surprise of millions of Americans that constipation is not listed as an indication for the use of laxatives. The first thing we should realize is that there is nothing sacred about a daily b.m. Each person has his own cycle; and if nature is not interefered with, that cycle will usually have manifested itself with amazing regularity in the person's early years so that by the time he reaches adulthood, he usually knows what his uninterfered-with pattern should be. Bowel movements no more frequent than once a week may not be abnormal if that has been the person's regular pattern for years. They certainly are not an indication for the use of laxatives.

In all fairness to the bowel mystique, it should be noted that purgation has for centuries been a cure-all for many ills, even in those people for whom daily regularity was not an end in itself. For many years, the concept of intestinal toxins was prevalent. This held that noxious materials were somehow formed in the bowel from the digested food products. If these "poisons" were then absorbed, the person would get sick in rather mysterious fashion. This theory has been totally discredited.

The trouble with the laxative habit is that it tends to be self-perpetuating. Certainly a person is not going to die a mysterious death if he feels the urgent need to take an occasional laxative. While its use is almost always not necessary, it will not kill him. The trouble is that laxatives work and therefore result in a relatively complete evacuation of bowel contents, even more complete than would normally occur under natural circumstances. As a consequence, the person's basic regular rhythm will be delayed for 2 or more days, leading the unwary into thinking they have once again become constipated and therefore require another laxative, and before you know it a psychic dependence as well as an intestinal dependence has occurred. In essence, why should the body exert its normal regular functions if this artificial chemical is doing the trick for it?

We now come to the occasional constipation that we are all subjected to, for example, when we travel. What should one do? Nothing. If, however, one feels from deep psychological needs, that something "just has to be done," then one might increase the roughage in one's diet and the fluid intake. Raw fruits and vegetables and bran products are good items for roughage, and at least the equivalent of eight glasses of fluid a day should be ingested. It is also important in persons who complain of constipation to establish a regular time for bowel evacuation. This should be followed conscientiously for, as one great philosopher put it, "Haste does not make waste."

There are times when the use of laxatives can actually be harmful. Anyone who has developed constipation because of a newly occurring abnormality or disease in his bowels should not use laxatives. They should never be taken for relief of an abdominal pain. They should never be taken by a patient who has cramps, colic, nausea, vomiting, or other symptoms of appendicitis. The death rate of patients with appendicitis who have taken laxatives before surgery is many times higher than among those who did not.

So, do not listen to the smiling, grey-haired mother as she tells you about the marvelous relief she has finally experienced with this new medication. The only mother to listen to is Mother Nature!

DIAPHRAGMATIC HERNIA

A hernia is an abnormal protrusion of a part of the body out of its normal postion. Thus the person with back trouble may have a herniated disc, which is a bulging of the cushioning pulpy material from between the vertebral bones where it belongs out to one side or another along the spine, frequently causing nerve symptoms if the bulge presses on a nerve. An inguinal hernia, which is most commonly seen in men, is the bulging down into the groin of intestinal parts which normally should stay in the abdomen.

What is a diaphragmatic hernia? What symptoms does it cause? And what can be done about it? Basically it is just an extension of the above principles of hernia, this time involving the diaphragm. The diaphragm is the large horizontal sheet of muscle going from the right to the left side of the body which separates the chest contents from the abdominal contents. This muscular sheet does have a few openings in it, however. Thus there is an opening for the aorta (the body's chief artery) to pass down from the chest into the abdomen where it gives off many of its major branches. Another important opening in the diaphragm is for the esophagus or gullet to go down into and join with the stomach.

This latter opening is the one we're interested in this time, for most diaphragmatic hernias occur there. What happens is that, for various reasons, part of the stomach bulges up through the diaphragmatic esophageal opening and can get "trapped" there, temporarily, by the normal contraction of the muscles that make up the diaphragm. Among the causes are the increased pressure of the abdominal contents due to obesity, pregnancy, or abnormal fluid in the abdomen. Some people seem to have a short esophagus so that the stomach seems to be pulled up into the opening. It is felt by many that there had to be an original weakness in the diaphragm muscles themselves or else the hernia would never have occurred in the first place.

An accurate idea of just how important the presence of a diaphragmatic hernia is may be difficult to arrive at since recent studies show that its presence can be demonstrated on X-ray, especially in older women, much more commonly than we used to think. The X-ray procedure is relatively simple: A solution of barium is swallowed in an attempt to outline the pocket (which sometimes can be a surprisingly large portion) of the stomach that protrudes up above the diaphragm. If a routine view doesn't show it, some radiologists will apply various forms of pressure bands over the external abdomen to see if they can pop any portion of the stomach up. Rarely, they will even tilt the X-ray table up so that the patient almost begins to stand on his head in an attempt to see if gravity will let the stomach move up.

The chief symptom is a pressure sensation or pain, in the mid-line, either low in the chest or high in the abdomen, depending on how you look at it. The discomfort of "funny feeling of fullness" usually occurs early after a meal—which is what one would expect since this causes the stomach to fill up and to "pop up." It can also occur if one lies down with a full stomach because gravity tends to push the stomach up. These people quickly learn that sitting up relieves their symptoms. The discomfort rarely lasts as long as an hour and is often relieved by belching or hiccuping since these procedures release the bubble of air usually trapped in the top of the stomach which, in turn, diminishes the full volume of the stomach and thus allows the herniated portion to slide down where it belongs. Sometimes the pain will go to the back, shoulders, and even down the arms, mimicking the pain of angina pectoris which is due to heart blood vessel disease. Such patients are usually quite happy to learn, after cardiograms and stomach X-rays have pinpointed the cause, that their problem is just a "hiatus hernia" (as a diaphragmatic hernia is also called) and not due to the heart.

One of the earliest symptoms is heartburn, especially after a heavy meal or lying down. This is due to the acid stomach contents regurgitating up into the esophagus and can usually be relieved by such simple measures as sitting up, drinking fluids, or taking an antacid. If the acid regurgitation is chronic enough to cause ulceration or burning of the esophagus, scarring may result and then the patient may have trouble swallowing, especially solid foods.

Occasionally a patient may have bleeding, either acutely or chronically, from a hiatus hernia. While an acute bleeding episode would be obvious by the loose, black, tarry stools, a slow chronic ooze might be manifested only by the symptoms of an otherwise unexplained anemia.

Finally what can one do about a hiatus hernia once it has been diagnosed (usually by various X-ray studies after swallowing a barium mixture)? The approach should at first be conservative: avoid overdistention of the stomach with food, take antacids regularly during periods of heartburn, and try to reduce the pressure in the abdomen by weight loss, if obesity is a factor. The next step would be to eat smaller than usual meals more often, with a tendency toward a low fat content since fat tends to slow down the emptying of the stomach. One should try to avoid food for at least 3 hours before going to bed. If necessary, one should go to sleep with the upper half of the bed elevated so that gravity can help keep the stomach down where it belongs.

An important but often overlooked piece of advice is to avoid tight bindings (such as tight corsets or tight belts) over the abdominal area, for the external pressure is quite easily transmitted internally with subsequent pushing up of the stomach through the widened hiatus.

These approaches will control the symptoms of most cases. When they fail, a surgical procedure to tack the stomach down under the diaphragm is often necessary and, when performed, is usually successful.

What we have learned through all of this is that surgery is not required unless medical treatment has failed, and certainly neither medical nor surgical treatment is required if the patient is completely free of symptoms and merely has the presence of a hiatus hernia on X-ray.

ULCER

For a reason that medical science has not yet been able to elucidate, peptic ulcers seem to be decreasing in frequency in the population of the United States. The ironic thing is that, after years of having so many peptic ulcer sufferers eventually have to come to the major surgery of removing parts of their stomachs, a new and very effective antiulcer medication has recently appeared on the medical horizon which may very well obviate the need for such major surgery in many ulcer patients.

Peptic ulcer really means two different diseases: Gastric ulcer and duodenal ulcer. Even though most people equate peptic ulcer with stomach ulcer, it is only the gastric ulcer that occurs in the stomach itself. The much more common duodenal ulcer really occurs in the first part of the small intestine which, of course, is not part of the stomach at all. Not only is the location of the two ulcerous conditions different, but even their cause and long-term outlook are often different.

Sweeping generalizations in any field often rest on shaky grounds; in medicine they may actually be dangerous to make; in the field of peptic ulcer, they may be downright wrong. Nonetheless, granting there will be many exceptions, the following concepts regarding the causes of peptic ulcers are generally accepted. The common form, duodenal ulcer, is almost invariably caused by an excess and prolonged secretion of stomach acid. It is true that the stomach lining itself has, in almost all people, sufficient protective mucus and chemicals to prevent much, or any, damage caused by the hydrochloric acid which it secretes as part of the digestive processes. Even though the duodenum and the pancreas secrete chemicals that help neutralize the acid that pours out of the stomach, a duodenal ulcer can nonetheless occur in those people with an excess acid production either because there is more acid being produced than can be effectively neutralized by those secretions or because the acidic fluid is bathing the very first portion of the duodenum just before the entry of the neutralizing chemicals. At any rate, since the duodenum does not possess the protective barrier against acid digestion that the stomach does, the constant bathing of it by acid can result in an eventual erosion which is called a duodenal ulcer.

Duodenal ulcers often occur in young people in their 20's. They seem to occur more often in men than in women. They often occur in people who seem to live lives subject to continual stress (real or imagined). Since alcohol is one of the prime stimuli to acid production, they occur quite frequently in those who abuse alcohol. Though smoking probably does not cause duodenal ulcers, the nicotine and other chemicals in the inhaled tobacco smoke do cause duodenal spasm, and many an unhappy possessor of a duodenal ulcer knows that smoking and having a relatively pain-free duodenum just don't mix.

Gastric ulcers are rarer than duodenal ulcers and are more mysterious. In many cases they are not caused by an excess of stomach acid; as a matter of fact, it is not unusual to find a lower-than-normal production of stomach acid in gastric ulcer stomach sufferers. Gastric ulcers tend to occur in an older population; and many a doctor is uneasy with, and follows very carefully, a person with a gastric ulcer to make sure that it heals in 6 to 10 weeks. In contrast to duodenal ulcers which rarely, if ever, become malignant, the occurrence of a gastric ulcer that doesn't heal promptly always raises the suspicion that it itself may be or is anatomically close to a malignancy.

Peptic ulcer is one of the few conditions in medicine where one can arrive at a diagnosis and a course of treatment almost entirely from the patient's story. So typical is that story for duodenal ulcer that one treats a patient for it even if the confirmatory X-rays are negative. As a matter of fact, if a person has a chronic, recurring story of upper abdominal discomfort occurring 4 or 5 hours after a meal or on an empty stomach, which is relieved by food or antacids, that person has, and should be treated for, a duodenal ulcer almost regardless of what his X-rays show. Since so many duodenal ulcers are followed by an X-ray visible scar, doctors have learned to treat the patient and not the X-ray. Thus, the finding of a duodenal scar on an X-ray picture may be merely evidence of an old healed ulcer and certainly does not warrant medical treatment unless the patient is currently having symptoms; and a patient with the appropriate symptoms should be treated regardless of the X-ray findings. This brings up the subject of X-rays. A G.I. (gastrointestinal) Series is an X-ray test which is very helpful in confirming the diagnosis of peptic ulcer. After the patient swallows, on an empty stomach, a thick barium-containing mixture, X-rays are taken of his stomach and duodenum as the barium goes through. Often, but not always, the test will outline the ulcer crater and the diagnosis is confirmed; but in at least 15% of what later have proved to be true peptic ulcers, X-rays did not show them. When the patient adds to the above story that the pain often wakes him at night from 2 a.m. to 3 a.m., almost the only tenable diagnosis is duodenal ulcer. Gastric ulcers often do not have this typical pain pattern. As a matter of fact, they are sometimes aggravated by food.

The mainstay of treatment of ulcers is to neutralize the acid. This can be done by attacking it directly through taking antacids, or indirectly by avoiding those foods or drinks which stimulate acid production. Though each patient will have to decide for himself exactly which items they are (and it is certainly true that in ulcers "one man's meat may be another man's poison"), the list of generally accepted items to be avoided by all ulcer sufferers is not too long: pepper, coffee, tea, cocoa, cola drinks, and alcohol. Smoking probably does not increase acid secretion but does cause spasm of the ulcer area. Besides antacids and diet, there are medications called anticholinergics which not only help decrease acid production but also help relieve spasm.

The revolutionary medicine of the past year or so is cimetidine which actually interferes with acid production and has been shown to greatly accelerate the healing of ulcers, thus avoiding the necessity of surgery in so many.

Surgery was not inevitable for all ulcer sufferers unless they ran into one of the major complications of a chronic peptic ulcer. These are generally considered to be only four: perforation of the ulcer through its wall which is an abdominal catastrophe and requires immediate surgery; significant or frequent hemorrhage from erosion of blood vessels in the ulcer area; obstruction to the passage of food out of the stomach because of the chronic scarring that has resulted from a chronic ulcer; or, finally, chronic intractable pain that goes on day after day, night after night, year after year.

It is the present medical hope, with the appearance of cimetidine and the mysterious decrease in ulcer frequency, that the occurrence of such drastic ulcer complications may begin to disappear.

My advice is simple. "Stop smoking. Avoid alcohol and highly spiced foods and coffee on an empty stomach. Other than that, eat what you want and can. If fried foods bother you, then *you* avoid them. If raw fruits bother you, then *you* avoid them. If nothing bothers you, then eat what you wish." There's no reason a person with a past history of ulcer must necessarily be sentenced to a lifetime of eating mush because he once had an ulcer.

GALLBLADDER

The gallbladder remains nowadays one of the few parts of the human body whose presence may not be important for the full and satisfactory function of the body. This statement is made with some hesitation since at one time the tonsils as well as the appendix were felt to be of not much current use to the body, and we now know that is not true.

Certainly, the gallbladder has a function: to concentrate the bile fluid which is concentrated by the liver. This concentrated fluid is then injected into the small intestine through the bile ducts, especially after mealtime, and serves an important function in the digestion and absorption of food. This function, however, does not seem to be in any way impaired in those patients who have had removal of the gallbladder. So, for now, it looks as if the gallbladder has no critical bodily function.

The production and flow of bile from the liver is important; otherwise, among other things, the digestion and absorption of most of the fats in our diet would be very seriously impaired. Also the absorption of Vitamins A, D, E, and K would be markedly diminished in the absence of the various complex acids and salts that make up the bile. But, to our present knowledge, none of these functions are in any way impaired if the bile is not concentrated.

The gallbladder is, however, an organ which can cause significant illness. One of the most common of these gallbladder diseases is the presence of gallstones. They may be even more common than doctors have realized. It was at one time felt that up to 10% of people would develop gallstones at some time in their lives. An interesting study has shown, though, that in the routine performance of autopsies, gallstones are found in the astonishingly high number of 20% of people.

Nobody really knows what causes gallstones. They're rarely seen in young people (except for those who have various hemolytic blood disorders where the red blood cells are being dissolved and broken down at such a massively accelerated rate that the excretory ability of the liver and gallbladder is exceeded, with the result that the red blood cell pigment forms heavy concentrations and can actually precipitate into pigment gallstones). Gallstones are more common in fat people than in thin people, and nobody knows why. They are more common in women than in men. The guess here is that there may be some obscure connection between female hormones and cholesterol, resulting in a higher content of insoluble cholesterol in women's bile fluid which eventually precipitates out as cholesterol-containing stones. This female hormone theory may also help explain why women who have had children have a higher incidence of gallstones than women who have never had children (because there is a great increase in female hormones during pregnancy).

Obviously, if 20% of Americans have gallstones, the great majority of gallstones cause no symptoms since most gallstone attacks, even mild ones, are not too common in our population. Among the mild symptoms of gallstones are: discomfort in the upper abdomen, especially after fried foods or certain vegetables. This discomfort can at times radiate to the back under the right "wing" at such times. Patients will also often complain of bloating and belching. It is obvious, however, that these are very common symptoms; and surely gallbladder disease cannot be suspected every time these occur. Rather, the pattern of repeated occurrences of these symptoms under essentially similar conditions should lead one to suspect that gallstones may be a factor.

The definitive way of making a diagnosis, of course, is by X-ray of the gallbladder with special dyes. The presence of gallstones is then generally easily detected.

The question arises: What to do if you find them? What can happen if they are not removed? One of the most serious and dreaded of gallstones complications is that one of these little stones can begin to travel out of the gallbladder into the relatively narrow passages leading into the small intestine and get stuck in one of these passages before getting into the intestine. This blockage will cause pain, fever, and jaundice, among other things. The patient becomes quite sick and, if the blockage persists, emergency surgery is in order (under far from ideal conditions).

Even if the stones sit in the gallbladder, they may be associated with attacks of acute cholecystitis (acute gallbladder inflammation) which, while less dramatic and drastic than the full blockage described above, still can make a patient very sick, often because bacterial infection sets in when a gallbladder has such stones in it on a chronic basis.

There is even a form of cirrhosis that can result from the prolonged presence of a gallbladder full of stones. On rare occasions a gallstone can erode right out of the gallbladder and cause various abdominal complications.

Another dreaded complication is cancer of the gallbladder. While a relatively uncommon cancer, it has been said that cancer of the gallbladder never develops in the absence of the chronic presence of gallstones. While one is always wary of absolutes in medicine, this belief is a fairly safe absolute. The cancer probably arises because of the chronic irritation the stones cause in the lining of the gallbladder.

Up until recently, the suggestion had been that everyone who has gallstones detected should have them removed by surgery because of the above-listed complications. There have been some medical dissenters to that opinion. The latter feel that: (1) gallstones are very common, (2) gallstone complications are not that common, and (3) the surgery required for gallstone and concomitant gallbladder removal is not always that innocuous. Certainly they do agree that people who are having repeated episodes of what sounds like gallbladder attacks, should have the stones removed if they are found. But what about the truly asymptomatic person in whom gallstones are found as the result of a routine medical examination? Some good medical opinion would have it that this latter group should be left alone.

During the past year or so, a radical new therapy has begun to be introduced: the taking of a medication by mouth to help dissolve gallstones. Still technically an experimental procedure, the first reports have come in positive in that success has been achieved in a significant number of cases whose gallstones are primarily cholesterol-containing. The drawbacks are that the medicine has to be taken daily for months, and perhaps even years, and in some cases it just doesn't seem to work. This medical therapy may turn out to be more acceptable than the previous "surgery for everyone" approach to the presence of gallstones in people who are completely asymptomatic.

9
Genito-Urinary

CYSTITIS

Granted that the most common of human *viral* infectious diseases are upper respiratory infections, it is not at all a well-known fact that the most common of human *bacterial* infections are those of the genitourinary tract. Of these so-called GU infections, urinary tract infections are by far the most common.

While those infections which affect the upper urinary tract, specifically the kidneys, are much more serious both in their acute symptoms and in the potential danger of their long-term complications, they are not so frequent as lower urinary tract infections, specifically cystitis. Cystitis is merely the medical name for inflammation of the urinary bladder. For reasons that are not known for sure, but which may be basically related to the obvious differences between the external anatomy of the two sexes, urinary tract infections, and especially cystitis, have been reported to be about ten times more frequent in girls and women than in boys and men. While it is believed that in very young children these infections can settle in the urinary tract area as a result of bacteria travelling through the blood stream or the lymphatic system, it is also true that, in older children and adults, the usual route of infection in cystitis is from the exterior inward to the bladder area.

The symptoms of acute cystitis are burning on urination or painful urination, the feeling of urgency of urination, and a subsequent increase in the frequency of urination. Also, there is often discomfort or even a low-grade pain either above the pubic area, or in the low back, or both. It is not unusual for patients to complain that they suddenly find that they are having to get up during the night to urinate. Blood in the urine may be noted (no one really knows why, but this symptom is more frequent in women than it is in men).

It should be mentioned in passing that not all GU infections are cystitis. If a person has chills, fever, nausea, vomiting, and a lot of high back pain, this usually represents a kidney infection. It is true that some kidney infections start out as cystitis, but this more dramatic picture of infection results because the infection has travelled upward to the kidneys from the bladder. Because of the potentially more serious complications, the speed and the extent of treatment is more urgent in kidney infections that it is in cystitis.

The diagnosis of cystitis is not a hard one to make. If one were to culture a sample of normal urine, few, if any, bacteria would be found. Since almost all cystitis represents a bacterial invasion of the lower GU tract, a urine culture in these cases usually reveals a massive growth of bacteria, usually more than 100,000 bacteria per milliliter of urine. Unfortunately, spurious diagnoses of cystitis have been made based on incorrect techniques of collecting the urine sample. The ideal sample collection is preceded by a cleansing of the external parts and then an actual "midstream" collection of the sample itself. The necessity of collecting a sample by catheterization is thereby obviated, which is a good thing in itself since, regardless of the scrupulous hygiene observed in the passing of a catheter, there is always the possibility that further infection may enter *via* the catheter itself.

The treatment of cystitis usually involves medication; however, if there is an anatomical abnormality which is causing a stricture somewhere along the exit passages from the bladder, then it will only be a matter of time before infection will recur. Therefore it is imperative that all such obstructions be corrected by surgical means.

In those cases in which no obstruction is present, a medical regimen which is continued long enough usually results in cure. Part of the medical regimen which is often ignored is keeping up an adequate fluid intake: One should drink at least eight glasses of fluid a day, be they in the form of water, coffee, tea, juice, milk, soft drinks, soups or whatever. There are various antispasmodics which have long been used to relieve the spasm of smooth muscle of the urinary tract;

there are also a number of medications which serve to relieve pain and discomfort in the area. While there is no reason why these should not be used, the mainstay of treatment of cystitis is antibiotics, sulfas, or other chemotherapeutic agents. (The list is too long to specify here.) Luckily, almost all cases of cystitis respond very satisfactorily to such a regimen. It is important that the therapy be continued for a week to 10 days, even though the symptoms subside long before that.

An ideal thing to do to insure that the infection has been eradicated, so that there is no fear of leaving behind a low-grade smoldering infection which can cause future problems, is to arrange for a repeat urinalysis 2 to 3 weeks after the patient has discontinued the antibiotic regimen. If that culture is completely negative and the symptoms are all gone, then so is the infection.

GU INFECTION

Infection is the most common disease of the urinary system. Usually mild and easily treatable, such infections can, however, be serious, if neglected, especially from the point of view of long-term complications.

Since some parts of the genitourinary tract, *e.g.,* the kidneys, lie quite deep in the body, one might expect that the majority of GU infections arise by bacteria being carried there by the blood stream. While such a path *is* one way, it is not so common as when infections come in from the outside and work their way up the GU tract.

Any structure along the GU tract can get infected but, in general, the deeper the structure involved, the more serious the infection. Among the parts that can be involved are (working from the outside in): the urethra, which is the final pathway for urine flow; the prostate gland, through which the urethra passes; the bladder, which stores the urine; the ureters, which are thin tubes which connect the bladder to the kidneys; and, finally, the kidneys themselves. Incidentally, it is probably the genetic length of the urethra in the male, as well as some possibly antibacterial properties of prostate secretions, that account for the fact that men have a much lower frequency of GU infections than do females.

The function of the GU system with its constant flushing through of urine is sufficient, in most cases, to assure that any organisms that might begin the journey up the tract are discharged before they really get a foothold. That is why it is imperative in any *recurrent* GU infection as well as all *severe* GU infections to investigate for any evidence of obstruction somewhere along the tract. Even minimal obstructions can lead to stagnation of the urine, and the urine is an excellent growth medium for all kinds of bacteria.

The classic symptoms of a GU infection are not always present in their full-blown manifestations. Urinary infections can sometimes be responsible for an individual's feeling "tired all the time" or a feeling of the "flu" that he can't shake. A woman with seemingly unexplained chronic low back pain or a child who begins wetting after having been toilet-trained may have such an infection. At other times the diagnosis will be almost obvious with frequent urination, a feeling of urgency along with burning, and pain on urination. The pain is sometimes mild, but it can be excruciatingly severe. Often there are chills and fever; and there may be nausea and vomiting, tiredness, and generalized muscle aching. Sometimes, the urine color will appear grossly abnormal, ranging from a cloudy, dark look to a frankly bloody appearance. There may be localized pain over the involved part; thus, back pain when the kidney itself is involved and suprapubic pain and tenderness when the bladder is involved.

When there is such localization of symptoms, the problem almost becomes obvious. In order to confirm it, your doctor will usually order a detailed urinalysis. The recent addition of special washing instructions to the patient before the actual urine is obtained has resulted in what is called "clean catch" urine specimens which are essentially as good for analysis as what would be obtained after passing a tube (called a catheter) into the bladder—and of much less discomfort to the patient!

The urine is then examined for white blood cells (pus cells), red blood cells and, most important of all, for the presence of bacteria. Sometimes bacteria are not visible on routine microscopic examination of the urine; in such cases, the urine is sent to a special laboratory for bacterial culture. There are a number of advantages to obtaining a urine culture even though it leads to a significant increase in diagnostic expenses to the patient. For one thing, a "negative culture," even though there were some bacteria seen on routine urinalysis, would raise the suspicion that those bacteria were just incidental contaminants and not really the cause of infection. On the other hand, a "positive culture" not only allows an exact pinpointing of what specific bacterium is causing the infection but, more importantly, it allows "sensitivity studies" to be performed which indicate what specific antibiotics will be effective against the invading organism.

Rarely, in those patients who fail to respond to medications, further diagnostic tests may be necessary. Special dye-injection studies of kidney X-rays may often locate the problem. Sometimes a cystoscopy examination is necessary, which involves the passage of an examining instrument up through the urethra to the higher reaches of the urinary tract.

Such detailed investigations of GU infections are necessary because the causative organism is usually of the "Gram-negative" type. Of the two large classes (Gram-positive and Gram-negative) of bacteria that are classified by their microscopic staining characteristics, most Gram-positive bacteria will be found in such conditions as boils, strep throat, and pneumonias, while most Gram-negative ones are found in urinary tract infections. The distinction is very important because some antibiotics are effective only against the Gram-positives; others are required for Gram-negatives. Thus, penicillin (one of the best of all antibiotics against Gram-positive bacteria) is usually ineffective for GU infections. Sulfas or the tetracycline antibiotics usually are quite effective.

Left untreated or inadequately treated, GU infections may have a subsidence of symptoms even though the infection is not completely eradicated. Thus, what started out as a simple cystitis (bladder infection) may over months or years ascend to the kidneys and cause a low-grade, chronic infection that can virtually destroy all normal kidney tissues. Since kidney damage is often a cause of high blood pressure, such patients may finally appear in their doctor's offices because of the symptoms and complications of their high blood pressure rather than because of the kidney infection that led to it.

A good but expensive piece of advice for anyone who's ever had a kidney infection is: Once it's all subsided and you've been off all antibiotics for at least 3 weeks, have a urine culture performed to make *sure* you're over the infection.

VENEREAL DISEASE

Despite the seeming worldliness and sophistication of our "emancipated youth," the increasing occurrence of venereal disease among them bespeaks a certain naivete or outright ignorance that can be dangerous—to themselves and others.

It's certainly true that the advent of antibiotics revolutionized the medical aspects of venereal disease, since antibiotics did more than just hold the diseases in check: They cured infected patients. However, antibiotics, if anything, may have aggravated the social aspects of V.D., since they may have resulted in a false sense of assurance that the problem no longer exists.

Whatever the responsible factors, the fact remains that venereal disease is now the country's leading communicable disease (or diseases—since when we speak of venereal disease we mean either gonorrhea or syphilis, which are by far the two commonest venereal diseases). Within the next 12 months, 1 million Americans will contract one or the other—which is a frightening statistic. Any other disease that attacked that many people would be considered an epidemic.

Partly responsible for this epidemic is the increase in sexual promiscuity, and also partly responsible is the lack of knowledge of what the diseases are.

It is probably categorically true that, with rare exceptions, the only way to contract a venereal disease is after sexual exposure to an infected person. There are only two exceptions I can think of: A newborn baby can develop a gonorrhea infection of his eyes if he passes through a birth canal infected by that organism; and a person may contract syphilis if he comes in close contact with any of the scattered moist patches in a person who has the secondary stage of syphilis.

Gonorrhea in the male is a less serious long-term disease than it is in the female because the signs and symptoms are more evident in men. First of all, knowing that he's recently had a suspicious contact will alert him to look for the signs which usually occur in 2 to 8 days after exposure. He'll have burning, pain, and frequency of urination associated with the passage of mucus which is at first clear, but which soon becomes profuse and greenish yellow. If he is treated adequately at this stage, the condition will clear up. However, if he ignores treatment, the infection can spread inwardly to involve the sexual passages and may cause sterility.

In the female, gonorrhea is potentially a more serious disease than in the male because very often acute symptoms are absent. There may be a discharge as in the male, but often this is mild, minimal, and of short duration. When the disease becomes chronic, it can have devastating consequences: Not only can it spread to involve the reproductive organs, but such severe abscesses can develop in the tubes that peritonitis may actually follow. Even if that doesn't occur, the scarring of the reproductive tract that can result from gonorrhea quite often leads to sterility. The treatment for gonorrhea is penicillin. At one time relatively low doses of penicillin were successful in eradicating it, but in recent years higher and higher doses have been required to eradicate organisms which seem to be developing a relative penicillin resistance.

Syphilis, the second of the major venereal diseases, can have even more widespread and lasting consequences. Again, because the areas involved are more easily visible, the symptoms and signs in the male are more easily detected than those in the female. The picture is, however, the same for both sexes. It begins as a chancre which is a painless, hard pimple which rapidly ulcerates. This is associated with enlargement of the lymph nodes that drain the involved area and is followed by a series of secondary lesions of the skin or mucous membranes. These secondary lesions are as infectious as the primary site. If the condition is still untreated, it enters a stage of quiescence during which infectivity is lost, so that one is no longer a menace to others, but the disease can continue its ravages internally in the patient himself. It can involve virtually any organ: It can strike the heart and cause a permanent leakage of one of the heart valves, which may eventually kill the patient; it can involve the bones; it can involve the brain and can cause a terrible form of deteriorative insanity. It can affect an unborn baby of a mother who is untreated and can cause its death or, if it is born alive, can result in permanent damage such as blindness and deafness.

Again the treatment is penicillin—in massive doses for the advanced stages. In both gonorrhea and syphilis, however, once the disease has spread to involve and alter the internal organs, treatment may halt the infection; but there is no return to normal of the damaged, scarred organs.

It has been suggested that *everyone* who is sexually promiscuous get a yearly blood test for syphilis. Even though the diagnosis may be made 11 or so months late, it can be cured (by plain old penicillin) in a few weeks—before permanent internal organ damage occurs (for with syphilis such damage takes longer than 1 year to develop). As for gonorrhea, the problem is more difficult. There is no blood test. If you wait too long, the discharge (in both sexes) may clear up before treatment is instituted; and the infection can then burn its way through the pelvic organs or urinary tract, leaving permanent damage and possible sterility in its wake. For a man, ignore no penile discharges after sexual exposure. For a woman, consider a culture test, regardless of symptoms.

How does one prevent V.D.? There is no vaccine in sight, so precautions should be exercised at each contact. The use of the condom should be emphasized. While it is not a 100% guarantee against getting V.D. (nothing is), it is very, very effective in preventing much of it. Some authorities suggest simple washing of sexual organs with soap and water both before and after contact and then urination as soon as possible afterwards. Again, this might help, but it's no 100% guarantee. The woman can also douche with certain preparations. Also, for the woman, feminine hygiene preparations, vaginal antiseptics, and contraceptive foams and jellies have something in them that combats gonorrhea and syphilis organisms. Again, only a help—no 100% guarantee.

The situation is bad because it's out of control. Maybe specific education will help remedy this. Maybe wide publicity to the problem will help. Maybe we *should* be giving free contraceptives to teenagers. No avenue should be left unexplored in combating this epidemic.

RENAL TRANSPLANTS

Kidney transplantation is one of the most dramatic medical "breakthroughs" of this century. There are numerous causes of irreversible kidney damage: Some persons are born with small kidneys which permanently lack the potential for normal growth; others may be born with a "horseshoe kidney" which is a fusion of the two kidneys with subsequent location in an abnormally low position in the body. Such kidneys tend to have a higher incidence of infection which, if uncontrolled, can lead to irreparable damage. Others may be born with polycystic kidneys which are kidneys riddled with fluid-filled cysts of all sizes which eventually cause very severe pressure damage to the kidneys. And there are other such congenital abnormalities that may eventually result in severely damaged kidneys.

A second large group of culprits in kidney damage are the various forms of nephritis. Glomerulonephritis (or Bright's disease) and pyelonephritis (which is a chronic smoldering infection of the kidneys) are among the leading causes here. These conditions strike an older age group: Bright's disease can follow any childhood or adult strep throat that is inadequately treated. (It is not, however, an actual infection of the kidneys with strep organisms.) Pyelonephritis can follow any inadequately treated kidney infection, at any age.

A third large group of end-stage kidney disease is found among persons who have severe forms of high blood pressure or arteriosclerosis—especially if these conditions have been present a long time. This third group, therefore, tends to be among older persons.

The one thing all these have in common is one extremely dangerous potential: end-stage kidney failure. Up until the mid-twentieth century, medicine had little to offer the sufferers of this condition. The toxic waste products of daily metabolism were accumulating in the blood instead of being excreted in the urine. These resulted in blood changes, heart changes, and even brain changes (for example, convulsions). Eventually, the patient died.

Then in the 1950's the concept of dialysis was introduced. By hooking up the patient's blood vessels, at great cost, to a very elaborate filtering apparatus, it became possible to filter, artificially, the waste products out of his blood. Unfortunately this process (which is still widely used) has a number of drawbacks: It is very expensive; it takes upwards of 12 hours to perform; and its effects last only a limited time, with repeated dialyses being required at least once a week and usually more often.

What seemed a revolutionary advance in this field was the introduction of kidney transplantation within the past 15 years or so. This actually involved the implanting of someone else's kidney into the patient by hooking it up to the blood vessels, while the patient's own diseased, nonfunctioning kidneys were either disconnected or actually removed.

This revolutionary approach, however, is not an unqualified success. Our bodies have vitally important "distant early warning systems": They are constantly on the alert to protect us from the invasion of our bodies by foreign proteins, be they viruses, bacterias, cancers, or somebody else's kidneys. What therefore results is a constant attempt (unfortunately, in this case, often successful) on the part of the recipient's body to reject this foreign matter (the transplanted kidney). Eventually drugs were developed which help suppress this defense mechanism of the body so that they allow it to tolerate the foreign substance, but the action of these drugs is *not* selective. They tend to allow for the tolerance of all foreign substances, including viruses, bacteria, etc. Naturally, the latter can cause serious infections, at times life-threatening in their own right. It is not unusual to see such patients die of overwhelming infection in the fact of a functioning kidney transplant.

A final development toward the perfection of kidney transplants involved using kidneys which were as antigenically close to the recipient as possible for the closer such kidneys resembled those of the recipient, the less would be the likelihood of rejection. A kidney from an identical twin would be ideal because it probably wouldn't be rejected at all. That from some other close relative also stood a fairly good chance of acceptance. Of course, there is a shortage of such available kidneys because closeness of relatedness does *not* insure that there is antigenic similarity between donor and recipient.

As a result, an elaborate series of tests have been developed to screen for antigenic likenesses so that the potential pool of donors could be enlarged. Already kidneys of the recently-deceased nonrelatives are being used.

All of which brings us to an article I have read. The author pointed out that in the not too-far-distant future, organ transplantation may become comparable to blood transfusions and "then the problem of donation from an unrelated living person will have to be faced." I read on, in some confusion. What problem? After all, I thought, if a living person wants to donate a kidney to a nonrelative and the antigenic match is good, so what? Well I soon found out that it isn't done. Such kidneys *won't* be accepted. The genetically unrelated living volunteer is now excluded!

Between 1964 and 1971, 60 such persons were allowed to donate their kidneys but not anymore. Why? "The genetically unrelated living kidney-donor volunteer, who comes forward and offers to donate one of his organs to someone in need who is unknown to him, has always been regarded with suspicion and distrust by the medical profession and is now barred altogether from donation." Suspicion and distrust? Why? Because they doubt his mental stability! It's almost as if, to put it bluntly, anyone who wants to lay down his kidney (not his life) for someone else must be crazy!

The article in question is a plan for a revision of such attitudes. Sure, the author recommends careful medical and psychological screening; sure, he insists it must be a free, informed choice on the part of the donor without coercion *in any form;* sure, the donor should be told that, even though it seems to be a good antigenic match, the transplant might still fail, or the patient might die of something else; but having been told this, he should then be allowed to make his donation if he wishes.

The author goes on to cite examples of seemingly normal people who have in the past been allowed to donate an organ. He quotes one summary study which found that:

The act of making such a gift becomes a transcendent experience, akin to a religious one. Many donors testify that giving an organ was the most important, meaningful, and satisfying act of their lives: one that increased their self-knowledge, enhanced their feeling of self-worth, gave them a sense of totality, belief, and commitment and increased their sense of unity with the recipient, people in general, and humanity.

In short, they were not metally disturbed!

Let's face it: There aren't too many people in this world who are about to volunteer anything of themselves (not even their money) to any stranger. But when we begin to look with an extremely jaundiced eye upon anyone who might (assuming that he's passed the test of not being mentally unbalanced), then I think we've come to a sorry pass indeed.

10

Infection

FOOD POISONING

Food poisoning is a nonspecific term which, from unpleasant personal experiences, means many things to many people. It can be caused by certain *chemicals* which are accidental contaminants of food but which in themselves are so toxic and irritating that we get sick. An example of this would be the much-publicized case of pesticide residuals contaminating grain which occurred in the Southwest. Another famous instance would be Minamata disease in Japan caused by extremely high levels of mercury in the local fish.

Another class of chemical food poisoning is caused by eating certain plants or animals which contain a naturally occurring poison. Examples of this would be the ingestion of poisonous mushrooms or some of the rare fish and shellfish poisons.

Then there are the infectious forms of food poisoning in which the cause is *bacterial* contamination. There are a number of forms of this of which some of the most well known are those caused by *Salmonella* (such as those illnesses recently associated with pet turtles).

Another form of bacterial food poisoning is that caused not so much by the multiplication of the contaminating bacteria as by a toxin that they produce. One such example is *Staphylococcus* toxin food poisoning (the kind so frequently associated with poorly refrigerated cream-filled pastries), which tends to make us very sick *in* a short time but, luckily for us, *only* for a short time.

A third form of bacterial toxin food poisoning is the one to which the rest of this article will be devoted. It's a name to strike fear even in the hearts of the fearless: botulism. Fortunately, botulism is a very rare disease, and perhaps its very rarity is responsible for the widespread publicity it gets when it strikes.

The bug responsible for botulism belongs to that totally unpleasant family of bacteria which include the organisms responsible for tetanus and gas gangrene. *Clostridium botulinum* (as the botulism bacterium is called) comes in six strains: A, B, C, D, E, F. F is very rare, and C and D cause disease only in animals. A, B, or E, however, produce some of the most potently toxic-to-humans poisons known to man. It has been estimated that fewer than 10 ounces of botulinum toxin, properly distributed, could kill every man, woman, and child *in the world.*

The botulinum spores are soil dwellers, being found all over the world. Type A spores are common in the western United States, whereas B spores are found in the eastern United States and Europe. Type E (the one usually found with fish-borne botulism) is found in northern latitudes, often being isolated from lakeshore mud, coastal sand, and sea-bottom silt.

These bacterial spores are all killed by exposure to moist heat at 120°C for 30 minutes. The toxins produced by the spores are even more heat sensitive, being destroyed by boiling 10 minutes or by exposure to 80°C for 30 minutes. Nevertheless, human disease still occurs often enough to indicate that these relatively simple precautions are not always followed.

What causes human poisoning is not so much the ingestion of the bacteria as it is the ingestion of the toxin they have been producing in the contaminated food prior to its being eaten. A large variety of home-processed foods, and recently, to great publicity, some commercially processed products have been implicated in outbreaks of botulism in the United States.

Food contaminated with A and B botulinum strains may often appear spoiled because of some special enzymes produced by these bacteria. However, many Type E bacteria do not produce these enzymes, so that foods containing Type E toxin may appear and taste perfectly normal. A and B toxins are absorbed from the stomach and upper small intestine and are resistant to digestion by the enzymes of the gastrointestinal tract. The disease itself, botulism, may vary from a mild indisposition that requires no medical attention to a rapidly fatal disease terminating in death within 24 hours. Usually symptoms begin 12 to 36 hours after the contaminated food is eaten.

Weakness, dizziness, and unusual tiredness are often early symptoms. While nausea and vomiting may be severe with Type E disease, they are less frequently observed in cases of A and B intoxication. There is often a severe dryness of the mouth and throat, sometimes even with pain in the throat.

The dreaded neurological symptoms may occur early or may be delayed for 12 to 72 hours. They include blurred vision, double vision, difficulty in speaking and swallowing, and muscle weakness. When the respiratory muscles become involved, difficulty in breathing ensues. The mind remains clear throughout, and usually there is no fever.

Most patients with botulism die of respiratory failure. Thus, an artificial lung may prove to be life-saving. Enemas are given to remove any unabsorbed toxin from the large intestine. If the patients are negative for serum sensitivity by skin test, antitoxin to A, B, and E should be administered. Unfortunately, in Type A poisonings, antitoxin probably doesn't alter the course of the disease once symptoms have developed. Antitoxin does seem to be quite helpful in Type E cases, even after onset of symptoms.

Mortality from Type A botulism is worst of all: 60–70%. With Type B it is 10–30%, and for Type E, 30–50%. However, if the patient survives the severe paralytic part of the illness, recovery is usually rapid and complete return to health can be anticipated.

COMMON COLDS

There are people who will swear that if they get their feet wet or their heads wet or get caught in a draft that they'll soon be catching a cold. There are others who feel that such beliefs are just a lot of folklore. What do medical studies reveal in this area? Well, for one thing, it isn't an area of overwhelming medical interest so that there aren't research laboratories all over the world frantically trying to find a solution. There have, however, been a few studies over the years investigating this area; and so far the medical results have come down on the side of the scoffers. No study has yet corroborated the impression that various forms of inclement weather exposure result in the common cold.

Personally, I still have a little reservation about the problem, but it's only a hunch, not based on any scientific observations. Nonetheless it might be worth reviewing what *is* known about catching infections so that we can put the problem in perspective.

The problem of becoming ill with an infectious disease is at least twofold:

1. Exposure to the infectious agent from the environment.
2. The level of the internal resistance to that infectious agent.

It is this second factor which is a highly variable one and which, therefore, makes blanket rules regarding infections impractical.

The first factor is obvious. One must have exposure to the infecting organism before one can get an infection. Even the "draft - wet feet" people admit that. Thus, if one has no significant viruses or bacteria in one's nose or throat and one is not exposed to anyone having such infectious organisms, then all the drafts in the world aren't going to cause an infection. Infections *always* result from the union of the bug and you. Without the bug, there's no infection.

Now we come to the much more complex second factor mentioned above: the level of internal resistance. It is well known, for instance, that one cannot get (except under most unusual circumstances) second attacks of measles, mumps, or chickenpox. Therefore, even if one were to come into intimate contact with a person infected with one of these viruses, the likelihood of one's contracting the infection a second time is extremely remote. These conditions are virus illnesses—as is the common cold. Although there is no absolute certitude in the matter, there seems to be some real medical evidence that, once a person has been exposed to a virus illness, he, more often than not, will have a lifelong immunity to that particular virus. The reason, therefore, that people keep getting influenza (which is a virus infection) is because the virus itself keeps changing. Also, there are so many "cold" viruses, all of which produce the same symptoms of sneezing, coughing, and runny nose that it may very well be true that even in the area of colds one doesn't catch the same virus twice.

There is more, however, to the problem of resistance than specific protection from previous exposure to that virus. It is fairly well accepted, medically, that once a person has fully recovered from a recent cold, a period of weeks, or even months, may go by during which his resistance to other "colds" is high even though some of the viruses he is being exposed to are new to him, and therefore, theoretically, ones to which he should be susceptible. The reasons for this resistance may have to do with certain blood constituents such as interferon and others, an area which will be discussed later in the article.

At least one other important factor in resistance to infection is a nonspecific one, the one that reflects various levels of hormones, especially cortisonelike hormones, in our bodies. Thus it is well known that when one is given cortisone for a medical reason for prolonged periods of time, one's resistance to infections tends to go down. The human body is making its own supply of cortisonelike hormones all the time, and the delicate balance of these hormones is also a nonspecific but nonetheless probably significant factor in determining resistance.

We know that the body makes extra cortisone in response to stress, and it may turn out to be here that folklore and medicine will meet. Thus, for those persons whose bodies react to cold wet feet or drafts as if these were stressful situations, there may be enough of an increase in cortisone output that it overcomes the body's defenses and an infection results. But this is pure speculation.

All we do know is that the patient must be, so to speak, "ready" for it before most infections develop. There might even be psychological factors operative, but this also is speculation.

As mentioned above, all colds are due to viruses—but not all viruses cause colds. Among the implicated viruses are rhinoviruses, adenoviruses, respiratory syncytial virus, ECHO viruses, etc. What they have in common is the fact that their range of infectivity is limited to the upper respiratory tract (nose, throat, sinuses, and the upper lung passages called the trachea and bronchi); they do not cause encephalitis (brain inflammation) or hepatitis (liver damage) or any other systemic symptoms, including gastrointestinal symptoms. (While there is some evidence that so-called 24-hour or 48-hour viruses with nausea, vomiting, and diarrhea are, indeed, viral illnesses, they are not caused by the usual viruses that cause colds.)

Perhaps the most important therapeutic fact about viruses is that they are viruses—which is to say they are parasites, living on the products of the cells of the host they invade. Unlike bacteria, they do not possess their own separate metabolic cycles; therefore, viruses are not affected by metabolic inhibitors—which is what antibiotics are. Stated simply, it is an unpleasant truth that viruses are not affected at all by antibiotics and that the administration of antibiotics to treat the common cold, while it may make the patient feel that something significant is being done for him, is in actuality, ineffectual!

Now, while this is bad enough news to those who for years have been relying on antibiotics for their colds, the worst is yet to come: Aspirin and various aspirin-containing compounds do not help cure and get rid of the common cold. Certainly they help lower the temperature, they relieve achey feelings and headache—but they do nothing whatsoever to shorten the course of the illness itself. As a matter of simple fact, there is no drug known to medicine that will shorten the course of viral colds!

If antibiotics and aspirin compounds don't shorten the duration of a cold, then what should one do for it? Apropos of that, there's the old saying that "if you don't take anything for a cold, it'll last a week; if you take medicines, it will last 7 days." Generally, most doctors will agree with that, but there's some evidence that might have us modify it thus: "If you don't take anything for a cold, it'll last 5 days; if you do take medicines, it may last 7 days." Specifically, the ingestion of aspirin to lower temperature is under question here. Less than 10 years ago, a very interesting study was conducted in France on children with colds. Those with rectal temperatures of over 102.5°F were excluded (because such a fever is associated with enough discomfort that the specific lowering of such a fever by aspirin is desirable). However, it should be recalled that, generally, it is most unusual for a person with a common cold to run a temperature as high as 102.5°F. The French researchers then divided the children into one group which was given aspirin regularly to help normalize the temperature and a second group which was not given any medicine but in whom the cold was allowed to run its course. The surprising result was that the untreated group got well in 5 days while the treated group took 7 days to recover. The explanation advanced was that the slight fever seemed actually to be beneficial to those not given temperature-lowering medications. There may be a good amount of truth to that since viruses, being parasites, usually are adapted to very specific host environments, and a virus that can live happily at 98.6°F may very well die unhappily at 100.6°F. It seems that the body knows what it's doing after all.

Well then, what *should* one do if one has a cold?

1. Bed rest. Though this is a nice safe recommendation, it is somewhat impractical. Most people have 3–4 colds a year; and if they took to their beds every time they had a cold, we'd be an almost bed-ridden nation. (Allowing 1 week per cold, and 4 colds a year, we'd all be spending upwards of 1 month in bed a year.) However, when temperature is over 100°F, bed rest should be resorted to.

2. Call your doctor. Again, many may object to this as impractical ("my doctor's a busy man and, anyway, all I have is a cold"), and in part they may be right. But, if there's enough fever to take to one's bed, then one should call the doctor if only to have him make sure no more serious complications have set in. Seeing one's doctor early is especially important for the very young, the very old, those with any chronic diseases (such as liver or kidney disease), those with diabetes, those with any chronic heart or lung disease, and anyone with a past history of rheumatic fever.

3. Eat what you feel like eating, but in general avoid foods you have found particularly difficult to digest. If you don't feel much like eating solids, at least keep up your fluid intake. Not only does this help keep body temperature controlled, but it also serves to keep upper respiratory secretions loose and therefore aids in their expulsion.

4. Do not use nose drops—at first. Attempts to lessen secretions and improve nasal airway are not recommended in early stages of a cold. Later on, however, when secretions have thickened, nose drops are often helpful if used sparingly (not more than 3–4 times a day), not only in relieving symptoms but also in promoting sinus drainage.

5. Use a cough medicine—especially in the early stages when a dry, hacking cough which is not productive of sputum is present. Such coughs often interfere with sleep, and rest is important in colds. Once the cough is loose and productive, a cough

medicine should not be used. The quicker lung secretions are expelled, the sooner one feels better.

6. Do take aspirin if the aches and pains of a cold are bothering you. Do take aspirin if you have a bad headache. Do take aspirin if fever over 102°F is really "knocking you out." Do not take aspirin just because you have a fever. Fever (under 102°F) is not necessarily bad.
7. Unless your cold is due to an allergy, don't bother taking antihistamines. Antihistamines do not affect infections.
8. Do not—ever—take antibiotics that you just have lying around. And don't be disappointed if your doctor doesn't prescribe antibiotics. They don't do anything to a common cold anyway.

Something very special happens in the human body after a virus infection, such as a common cold. Not only is the specific infecting virus destroyed by the body's buildup of antibodies against it, but there is a secondary nonspecific beneficial effect of virus infections in general. In the past 15 to 20 years, a new body chemical, called interferon, has come up on the medical horizon. Interferon is a chemical which helps the human body combat virus infections in general. Its production is triggered by a preceding virus infection and, once triggered, the body levels of interferon remain elevated for anywhere from 2 to 3 months to considerably longer periods. It may be this interesting fact that accounts for the well-known observation that some people having much exposure to others with bad colds will not be infected, while other people, with similar exposure, will catch the cold. The virus itself probably has a uniform infectivity but, if it is visited upon us when our interferon levels are high, we just don't catch it. This varying level of interferon may explain another big fact about the common cold. Some of us will feel a cold coming on and then are rather pleasantly surprised to find it gone in 1 or 2 days instead of its usual week or so duration. It may be that the cold arrived when our interferon level was low enough to allow the virus to get in but high enough to prevent the virus from exercising its full sway.

Now we are in the realm of pure speculation. When one considers the marvelous condition of the human body's machinery, one is constantly impressed by the intricate degrees of protection found there; and this impression is based only on the relatively scanty amount of facts that medical science has elucidated about the body. Who knows what other delicate, finely balanced control mechanisms are yet to be discovered? We have evolved to such a high point of mechanical so-phistication in our bodies that I think one can safely say that every-one's normal situation is one of health and that disease is luckily a rare upset of the finely tuned body. There are so many disease con-trol mechanisms built into us! It has been estimated, for example, that the human body may destroy upwards of 100 cancers a day, so efficient is the internal mechanism towards maintaining health. If all that is true, as it seems to be, then why can't we seem, as an organism and a species, to be able not to catch common colds? And that set me to wondering: What if the common cold is an environmental neces-sity, a biological necessity so to speak, that we require in order to stay healthy in the long run? What if that annoying week of discom-fort is necessary to trigger interferon and perhaps other body chemi-cals that we don't even know about?

We have all read, especially in the past few years, of the possibility of a viral cause for cancer. Even if not a true virus in the sense that most of us mean by infective viruses, what if the cancer stimulant may be some viruslike altered protein that our body must recognize as foreign and thus destroy in order to keep healthy? Who of us would not wish to have as many common colds as possible in order to stimulate the necessary interferon or other chemical level that would protect us from such a dread disease as cancer? Isn't it wise of the body-environmental milieu to have had this interferon-stimulat-ing mechanism triggered by something as trivial as the common cold. Woe would indeed betide us if the trigger were only serious viral ill-nesses, such as measles, mumps, chickenpox, or smallpox!

It may be a good thing that medicine has not been able to come up with any kind of specific cure for the common cold. It may be that the very symptoms of the cold, such as low-grade fever and increased mucus production, are part of the interferon triggering mechanism. We just don't know. We may in the long run be doing ourselves a disservice in the control of cold symptoms if those symptoms are in-deed such protective-mechanism triggering factors. An interesting fact in the medical literature recently is that there are some unfortu-nate persons who are born with congenital deficiencies of their im-mune mechanism. Not only do they have increased susceptibility to viral infections in general, but they are unable to build up any kind of lasting immunity to viral infections. These people, therefore, lack the protective mechanisms that the common cold, for example, constantly resupplies us with. The frightening fact is that these young children are victims of various cancers at remarkably younger ages than would have been expected, if at all. This is not to say that the only cause of cancers are viruslike invasions, but those who have trouble in building up their body's virus combating mechanisms have trouble protecting themselves against cancer.

Man's frantic search for the cure for the common cold may indeed be a wild goose chase; for if he succeeds we might all be dead ducks.

FEVER SORES

Although fever sores often do crop up or, more likely, recur during periods of fever (in the "old days" when doctors saw a lot more pneumonia cases than they do now, it was more often than not the rule to see a crop of fever sores blossom, usually when the pneumonia itself was subsiding), their occurrence or reoccurrence does not require the presence of fever. Nowadays one sees fever sores most often as a result of exposure to sun, usually to too much of it.

It is not generally realized that all fever sores are the result of an infection right there at the spot of the fever sore. The underlying cause is, unfortunately, a virus rather than a bacterium. "Unfortunately" because if fever sores were bacterial infections, there would almost certainly be an antibiotic available that would lead to their quick eradication. However, fever sores, in common with just about every other infection caused by a virus, are not susceptible to any antibiotic. Millions of antibiotics are wasted regularly on people who just have a viral cold, but people demand them because they realize that a cold is an infectious disease. If they realized that fever sores were also infections, they probably would be demanding useless antibiotics for that also, thus exposing themselves to many of the side effects, and getting none of the advantages, of antibiotics.

The causative virus of herpes simplex (the medical name for the "cold sores" or the "fever sores," which are the most common manifestation of infection with this virus) is peculiar among viruses in that, generally, once you get it, you never get rid of it—even though there may be long stretches of seemingly virus-free intervals. Almost everybody contracts herpes simplex infection during the course of a lifetime, usually in one's younger years. It is, however, distinctly unusual for the infection to occur in an infant of fewer than 6 months of age because the antibodies against the virus from the mother's blood often linger that long in the baby. But, once that period is past, we're all ripe for herpes.

In most cases, however, the primary infection is mild or totally inapparent. Then the thing peculiar to the herpes virus occurs: It doesn't really go away but, rather, lies dormant—usually localized to the same area of skin where it manifested itself before. Generally, the involved areas are around the mouth, producing the well-known "fever blisters" or "cold sores." Pain often precedes the reappearance of the sores by 1 or 2 days, may last throughout the time of their presence, and may, rarely, actually increase in intensity after the lesions are gone.

The typical appearance of the recurrence is of a group of tightly-packed, clear blisters surrounded by a base of reddened, swollen skin. The most common location is on the lips at those spots where the skin of the lips joins the pinkish mucous membrane part of the lips. But they can occur on the chin, the nose, the cheeks, and even the ears.

The blisters soon rupture, oozing a clear, sticky, occasionally even slightly bloody fluid which then forms a yellow crust. So long as they do not become secondarily infected by bacteria, the lesions usually heal without scarring in 2 to 7 days.

Theoretically, if the stimulus (for example, exposure to sun) is sufficiently intense, almost everyone would experience recurrence of herpes simplex. Actually, susceptibility to their recurrence varies from individual to individual. Often worse in fair-skinned people, it may be so bad in some that they cannot even tolerate short exposures to sunlight or heat. Other persons have recurrences following short episodes of fever, common colds, minor gastrointestinal disturbances, or even unusual exertion. Pregnancy, menstruation, or even emotional strain may trigger an episode.

After all this, what can you do for it? Stay with us as we now glide into the mysterious but interesting realm of witchcraft, folklore, superstition, and scanty medical facts. Everyone knows what to do for fever sores (unfortunately, almost everybody has a different cure for them). "Use camphor, any form of camphor," say the grandmothers in the audience and they may be right. "Alcohol, 70% alcohol," the grandfathers in the audience say—and they may be right—for that too seems to work. Most everybody agrees that moisture aggravates the condition—so moist soaks are out. However, I've come across at least one medical textbook that says wet dressings may be necessary. So there!

What else is there for fever sores? Lots: some recommend calamine lotions; still others swear by tincture of benzoin. Many feel (and I tend to agree) that a sun screen lotion applied before each exposure to the sun will either keep them from appearing or keep them down to a mild flare-up.

The old witch doctor remedy of giving a person a smallpox vaccination to prevent fever sores probably is as useless as giving antibiotics for a fever sore once it has appeared. Most doctors stay clear of cortisone preparations because they potentially can make the disease spread.

For the overwhelming majority, tincture of time is all that is needed before the whole thing goes away. Unfortunately, most of us can't "grin and bear it" because when we grin, it hurts.

GERMAN MEASLES

Because the German measles vaccine is now a reality, thousands of pregnant women throughout the country are able to breathe easier.

Vaccines are important, because to date they represent medicine's most effective weapon against many viral illnesses. In contrast to bacterial illnesses (such as most pneumonias, kidney infections, and infected wounds) which are almost universally susceptible to one or more of the many antibiotics now available, virus infections are almost universally *resistant* to all antibiotics. Unfortunately for man the great majority of his illnesses are viral in nature: from such relatively minor afflictions such as the common cold and influenza to the much more severe viral illnesses such as hepatitis, polio, yellow fever, and smallpox.

We all know, however, that we *do* have protection against many of these antibiotic-resistant illnesses. Smallpox and yellow fever are virtually unknown today in the United States and, thanks to Salk and Sabin, polio is rapidly joining their ranks. How has this protection been achieved? Vaccines—which are live or killed altered virus particles injected into well people so that subsequent exposure to that particular virus does not result in disease.

The problem with vaccines is much more complex than with bacterial infections. In bacterial infections, one treats *one* person when he is ill. In vaccinations against viral infections, one has to treat hosts of people when they are well so that they won't ever get the virus in question (for once they get a viral illness, medicine rarely has any specific cure).

Why bother treating a lot of well people for such things as the common cold and influenza? After all, they are not very serious conditions in themselves. But they do result in untold hours of personal misery and financial loss. As to smallpox, yellow fever, and polio, well, very few people need to be convinced to obtain protection against them.

Where does German measles fit into this spectrum? After all, isn't German measles (or rubella as it is called technically) really "3-day measles" which is relatively much milder than "real measles"? Yes, it is. Generally the German measles patient is uncomfortable for a few days and then gets well quickly. If only to avoid 3 or 4 days of such illness, it would be worth trying to obtain a vaccine against the German measles virus. But the picture is more complex with German measles.

In the early 1940's reports first appeared from Australia and have since been confirmed all over the world that German measles in a pregnant woman is a very serious illness indeed—not so much to her as to her unborn child who may, as a result of the mother's having this relatively "benign" infection during the first 3 months of her pregnancy, be born with various congenital abnormalities. As the years have passed, the percentage of involved babies has diminished from an originally feared 80–90% to the present 10–20%, but that hard core of 10% or so remains. Giving birth to a child with a congenital abnormality is a very serious problem indeed.

Though there is no cure for German measles, medicine has had one tool against it: gamma globulin. The prompt injection of large amounts of it into any pregnant woman exposed to German measles in her first 3 months of pregnancy has generally been successful in preventing the subsequent birth defects. Of course, if the mother is sure she has already *had* German measles before her pregnancy, then no precautions are needed at all because she can't catch German measles twice. As a matter of fact, one medical approach has been the recommendation that *all* girls be deliberately exposed to German measles before reaching puberty.

It is because of this background that the announcement of a successful vaccine against German measles aroused much enthusiasm. The vaccine has been so perfected that, in contrast to the "regular measles" vaccine where the inoculated person may often get a mild transient form of the disease, the German measles vaccine gives immunity against German measles (only) without causing symptoms in almost all those inoculated.

HEPATITIS

Although hepatitis is a relatively uncommon disease, its occurrence among adults is certainly more frequent than it was 20–30 years ago. One particular form of hepatitis—serum hepatitis—has achieved notoriety because it's the hepatitis that occurs in drug addicts. Since the disease is potentially serious, a brief review of some facts might be in order.

Just as appendicitis means inflammation of the appendix and laryngitis means inflammation of the larynx or voice box, so hepatitis means an inflammation of the liver (*hepar* means liver in Latin). Specifically, however, hepatitis refers to an *infectious* inflammation of the liver. The infecting agent in hepatitis is a virus, not a bacterium; therefore we know right off that antibiotics will not cure the disease.

There are at least two strains of hepatitis virus, the chief of which are virus A which causes infectious hepatitis and virus B which causes serum hepatitis. Although one can't tell under the microscope which is the causative virus in a specific case of hepatitis, the way the disease is caught and the long-term aftereffects of the disease differ for the two virus strains, so that very often doctors have a pretty good idea from the overall picture which of the two forms of hepatitis they're dealing with.

Infectious hepatitis is by far the commonest form of the disease. At one time it used to be a very common disease of childhood; but now, with better sanitation and diminution of overcrowded living conditions, many persons can get through childhood without ever contracting hepatitis. Just as in the case of polio, hepatitis in childhood is usually a very mild disease while in adults it can be a very serious one. It is the increasing frequency of infectious hepatitis among *adults* that has made many persons aware of the condition in the first place.

Basically, infectious hepatitis results from the ingestion of virus excreted by an infected person—either directly due to poor sanitary and hygienic conditions, indirectly through such agents as contaminated milk or water, or even through an intermediary such as the ingestion of contaminated shellfish which have concentrated the virus from a polluted seawater environment. A few epidemics along the East Coast have been traced to the ingestion of poorly cooked clams (raw clams from contaminated areas are *absolutely* to be avoided; even steaming the clams is not sufficient protection—unless one continues to steam the clams for 9 minutes after the shell has opened. Fried clams are all right).

While infectious hepatitis is contracted orally, serum hepatitis (virus B) is usually contracted after innoculation. The passage of virus-contaminated blood from one infected person to a noninfected person is the usual way you can get virus B (although, theoretically, if one received a transfusion of blood from a virus A-infected person during the height of his infection, one would then have contracted virus A by inoculation rather than by mouth). Blood transfusions are the principal vehicles for virus B serum hepatitis, although the contaminated syringes of addicts are a more dramatic vehicle. On occasion inadequately sterilized dental and surgical equipment has been implicated, while contaminated tattoo needles are a notorious source of serum hepatitis.

Both conditions can cause yellow jaundice, dark urine, light stools, and enlarged, tender liver—all signs of liver involvement—along with more conventional signs of illness such as fever, weakness, loss of appetite (for food as well as loss of taste for cigarettes), headache, and muscular aches and pains. Treatment consists of bed rest, careful dietary management, and, rarely, cortisone compounds.

Even though most patients recover completely, there can be complications in others. Rarely, it is very rapidly fatal; it can become chronic and can even progress to cirrhosis with all *its* complications. Some authorities believe that complications follow serum hepatitis more frequently and seriously than infectious hepatitis.

In short this is a disease to avoid if possible. If one has been exposed to virus A infectious hepatitis, taking specially pooled gamma globulin protects against or at least modifies the disease. Until recently it was felt that gamma globulin offered no help in virus B serum hepatitis, but some new studies indicate that a special hepatitis B gamma globulin may be helpful in such cases.

Although the disease can be very serious, one should keep it in perspective by recalling that about 99% of persons with it have and get over it completely without any long-term damage.

IMMUNIZATIONS

We should remember that, with few exceptions, there are no really effective vaccinations against infections caused by bacteria. Thus one does not get "shots" to protect one against strep throats or bacterial pneumonias. The few exceptions in which shots *can* protect against bacterial illnesses are very important, though.

1. Cholera is caused by a bacterium, and shots should be given to travelers who are going to South and Southeast Asia as well as the Middle East. However, immunity lasts, at the most, 6 months, at which point a booster is needed.
2. Diphtheria protection should be offered to everyone, regardless of where they live. Luckily the immunity lasts for at least 10 years.
3. Tetanus or lockjaw shots are something most people are aware of and quite willing to get. They also should be given to everyone and, as in diphtheria shots, immunity lasts at least 10 years.
4. Pertussis or whooping cough shots should be given to all children because it is an especially severe illness in them. Those beyond age 6 who have never been immunized do *not* need to be since the disease is much milder in the older age groups.
5. Plague protection should only be offered to persons going to Southeast Asia or whose occupations bring them in contact with wild rodents. Immunity is not long-lasting, however; and booster shots should be given once or twice a year as long as exposure persists.
6. Typhoid fever used to be a prevalent killer in the United States, and at one time protective shots used to be recommended for all

persons. This is no longer necessary. The shots should instead be reserved for persons who are household contacts of known typhoid carriers, for all persons in areas when there are community or institutional outbreaks (such as in nursing homes or orphanages), and for those who are traveling to areas where typhoid fever is so prevalent that it is accepted as one of the area's "background illnesses." Typhoid fever shots are no longer recommended for persons going to summer camp. The period of protective immunity is intermediate between those we've considered above: Under conditions of continued or repeated exposures, a booster dose should be given every 3 years.

(Finally, and to be mentioned only for the sake of completeness, paratyphoid shots, which used to be routinely given along with typhoid shots, are no longer to be used. Not only had their efficacy never been proven, but recent trials have actually shown paratyphoid shots to be ineffective in offering protection. Besides, the giving of them results in an increase in vaccine reactions.)

The above are the only bacterial-caused conditions for which any kind of really effective immunization procedures are available. There is one more condition which is caused by an organism smaller than a bacterium but larger than a virus for which immunization procedures are also effective. The only rickettsia-caused infection for which vaccination is generally recommended is:

7. Typhus, a louse-borne disease which has become increasingly uncommon with the worldwide application of insecticides and the generally improved standards of living. However, the disease is still prevalent in many areas of the world; and vaccination is indicated only for travelers going to such areas. Immunity is not long-lasting, and boosters every 6 to 12 months are needed.

The list of immunizations concludes with those vaccinations that are intended as virus disease prophylaxis.

1. Smallpox has been one of the most dreaded diseases known to mankind, spreading its history of terror at least as far back as

the second century A.D. In one 18th century English epidemic, it accounted for over 30% of *all* the deaths of children at that time. In a Boston, Massachusetts, epidemic in 1752, 30% of all residents contracted the disease, and over 30% of them died of it!

In England, in 1721, one of mankind's greatest discoveries against infectious diseases occurred. We don't know who first thought of it, but it was discovered that the deliberate, controlled inoculation of the smallpox material (they didn't know in those days that it was caused by a virus; as a matter of fact, in those days they didn't even know what a virus *was)* into the unexposed recipient protected him against the natural disease. Unfortunately, they were inoculating people with the smallpox virus itself; as a result, 1 to 2% of those vaccinated died, but in a real way that was better than 30% dying if the disease struck in its usual course.

Then, in 1798, Jenner of England reported that if the virus of cowpox (rather than smallpox) was used to inoculate susceptible persons, it afforded them protection against subsequent *smallpox* exposures. This vaccinia virus did not, however, lead to any *smallpox* complications because it was a different virus. This process of vaccination (derived from the name of the cowpox virus) became widespread as its safety was realized, and it was this which was being done to all of us who got smallpox vaccinations. (Incidentally, the word *vaccination* is correctly applied, technically, only to smallpox vaccinations, all others being either inoculations or immunizations.)

Now, along comes the great controversy. The United States Public Health Service, on September 25, 1971, recommended the discontinuation of routine smallpox vaccination! How come? Has smallpox disappeared from the face of the earth? Practically! Then, what does it all mean?

The concept of vaccinating everybody against smallpox was introduced when smallpox was widespread and uncontrolled. At that time, it was so important to vaccinate susceptibles that it became a legal requirement, especially for people traveling internationally.

The reason for the recent change in recommendations is that in the United States and in most of the rest of the world, vaccination procedures have succeeded so well that smallpox is virtually nonexistent. Through the most wide-ranging Public Health efforts in the history of the world, smallpox has been completely eradicated from the world. In 1976, when this was first declared, there was general rejoicing and then some subsequent concern as a few isolated cases were still reported from the last stronghold of smallpox–Ethiopia. However, an intensification of Public Health efforts concentrated on Ethiopia has been so successful that no cases of smallpox have been reported from there so it does look as if smallpox is gone forever at last. Locally, even before the complete eradication of smallpox, the recommendations to discontinue smallpox vaccination in the United States had already been made since the disease was virtually unknown here; and the vaccine did cause, in very, very rare cases, some significant unpleasant side effects. We had reached the situation where the cure (the vaccine) was causing more trouble than the disease itself and so, except for people who are traveling to certain countries which still require smallpox vaccination (for rather difficult to explain reasons), smallpox vaccination is no longer administered to anyone in America.

Why not just continue vaccinating everybody anyhow? Because though they occur very, very rarely, there are varying degrees of complications associated with the vaccinations themselves. Therefore, the U.S. Public Health Service has decided that nonselective vaccination against smallpox unnecessarily exposes a large segment of the United States public to the risk of complications resulting from the vaccination itself–a risk greater than the probability of their contracting the disease.

The probability of contracting smallpox in the United States is extremely low and continues to decrease. There has not been a documented case of smallpox in the United States since 1949, and importation from another country is the only way in which smallpox could occur in this country. Importation into the U.S. is unlikely for two reasons: (1) Worldwide eradication efforts have brought about a significant decrease in the number of cases of smallpox; and, (2) in this country, there is a national surveillance system to identify suspect cases. Upon confirmation of a suspect case, there are efficient emergency procedures for managing the case and contacts and for preventing spread of the disease.

The new recommendations, therefore, are that vaccination should routinely be required only of people at special risk: that is, travelers to and from countries where smallpox may still exist and health services personnel (doctors, nurses) who come into contact with patients.

Many doctors are startled and somewhat leery at this reversal of one of the most time-honored of medical practices, and it will take a while before everyone gets on board. However, the public health decision was based on very careful statistical analyses and the opinions of many consultants.

2. Yellow fever is prevalent only in Africa and South America. Therefore, only those living or traveling there should be vaccinated. Protection seems to be excellent so that booster doses are recommended only once every 10 years.

3. German measles vaccination is one of the newest—and potentially most valuable—immunizations available. German measles itself is, of course, a relatively benign disease; but if a pregnant woman contracts it early during the course of her pregnancy there is a very real possibility of serious congenital abnormalities occurring in her unborn child. Anyone who has ever had true German measles (the so-called "3-day measles") is permanently protected against a second attack, and vaccination in these people, while doing no harm, would be superfluous. Vaccination in men is really not required either, for the infection in adults, though not so mild as in children, is still not a very serious one; and its effects on the unborn fetus apply only to women. All children between the ages of 1 and puberty should be vaccinated against German measles.

4. Polio is now a disease of the past. It's hard to realize that up to 10 or 15 years ago it was, perhaps next to smallpox, one of the most feared infections of all. Everyone should receive polio vaccination—it's as simple as that. The original "Salk shots" did not give lasting immunity and have since been largely discontinued, yielding to the three-dose oral Sabin series of polio doses. Because of the present rarity of the disease in the United States, vaccination of the previously unexposed (either via natural infection without residual effects or prior vaccination) is a

moot question. Most doctors feel it does no harm and would probably give it, especially to those adults traveling to those areas where polio is more prevalent than in the United States. The need for oral polio boosters is uncertain, and such oral boosters are being given if there is any uncertainty regarding the adequacy of existing protection.

5. Mumps vaccine is another of the recently introduced vaccines that will probably soon be universally given to children before they reach puberty. This will serve a double purpose: It will prevent mumps which can be a much more serious illness, even in children, than German measles; and it will prevent that 25% incidence of testicular damage and sterility that can occur if the infection involves a male beyond the age of puberty. For those who have had naturally-occurring mumps, no vaccination is required, for permanent immunity is conferred by the illness. For those adult males who are sure they have never had mumps, some doctors have suggested that it would be a good idea to receive the shot. Not enough time has elapsed to ascertain whether or not booster shots will be needed.

6. Measles vaccine is now another of the well-established, though relatively new, vaccinations. Regular measles, unlike German measles, is not known to produce any adverse effects upon the unborn child, but it can be quite a severe infection in itself and is thus worth avoiding. Measles vaccine is recommended for all children. At present no recommendations are made for vaccinating adults, since almost all adults over 15 years of age are immune. No booster doses are needed.

That covers the list of recommended vaccines against viral illnesses. A few words might be added about one other viral condition in which the picture is less clear-cut—influenza.

7. Influenza vaccinations protect only against infection caused by the specific strain of virus included in the vaccine. Unfortunately, unlike all the other viral illnesses listed above, influenza can be caused by many different variants of the influenza virus. Actually the virus just seems to change its basic structure every few years, so that an effective vaccine of a few years ago may no longer be effective, because of a viral change. So specific influ-

enza vaccinations are required whenever a new epidemic is in the offing.

SUGGESTED IMMUNIZATION SCHEDULES

There have been some recent outbreaks among preteenagers and teenagers of "childhood diseases" which everyone had assumed had been essentially brought under excellent control, if not completely eliminated, by the multitude of immunizations and booster shots to which our children are subjected. This led to intensive investigations to try to determine the reason, which turned out to be what we in America have taken for granted: the relative absence of these infectious diseases. We, therefore, are no longer "subjecting" our children to immunizations and boosters as much or as frequently as they should be.

When one recalls that measles can be fatal, that chickenpox can be a very serious disease, that diphtheria very often was fatal, that whooping cough often left the child with permanent irreversible damage to his lungs, that polio could leave a person crippled for life if it didn't kill him right away, one can rightly be astonished at the apathy of Americans in making sure that they and their families are protected against these potentially killing or maiming diseases.

The following is a chronological rundown of what you and your children should have received, in terms of immunizations. If part or all of the suggested regimen has not been administered, give serious thought to rectifying it.

Most normal children are begun on an immunization program before the age of 1 year. Thus:

2 months— The famous DPT shots are begun. The D protects against diphtheria, the P protects against pertussis, and T protects against tetanus. This is the first of a series of shots since, contrary to some public opinion, one shot *doesn't* offer adequate protection. Also at 2 months, the first of a series of trivalent oral polio virus vaccines is given to the child—by mouth, of course.

4 months—   The second shot in the series of DPT and the second oral polio material are given.

6 months—   The third of each is given.

1 year—   Now, either singly, or as combined vaccines, measles, mumps, and rubella (German measles) immunizations are given. Recently, the tuberculin skin test (one form of which is known as the Tine Test) has been suggested as an important adjunct at age 1. This tells the physician whether the child has been significantly exposed to tuberculosis and can be very important in determining whether treatment should be then offered to prevent any of the serious late-life complications that have caused the devastations of tuberculosis down through the centuries.

1-1/2 years—   A booster of DPT and oral polio is given again.

4–6 years—   The final dosage of DPT and oral polio is given.

14–16 years—   An adult type tetanus and diphtheria toxoid booster is then administered at a 10-year interval from the previous booster and continued every 10 years thereafter throughout life (see below).

For those children who were not immunized in infancy, the following schedule is recommended.

If they are 1 through 5 years of age:

1st visit—   DPT, oral polio, and tuberculin test.

1 month later—   Measles, mumps, and rubella immunization.

2 months later—   DPT and oral polio.

4 months later—   DPT and oral polio.

6–12 months
later or
preschool–   DPT and oral polio.

14–16 years–   Tetanus-diphtheria toxoid every 10 years.

Unfortunately, as recent investigations have shown, there are children who are 6 years of age and over who have not yet really had primary immunizations. For these children the following recommendations are made:

First visit–   TD (this is tetanus-diphtheria; the pertussis-whooping cough part is omitted because over the age of 5 whooping cough is much less serious than under the age of 5), oral polio, and tuberculin test.

1 month later–   Measles, mumps, and rubella immunization.

2 months later–   TD and oral polio.

6–12 months
later–   TD and oral polio.

14–16 years–   TD and every 10 years thereafter.

The above flow charts, if followed for every child in America, would really result not only in diminished frequency of these illnesses on a national basis–but would serve specifically to protect your child.

What about adults? It is estimated that most adults will have had these immunizations or the specific diseases in question sometime before they reach adulthood. The above schedule for children of 6 years of age and over is not one that should be followed by adults. Rather, a review of one's past immunizations and illnesses should be conducted individually with your doctor to determine which, if any, of the immunizations are in order for you. Many physicians do believe that an adult polio immunization series is a good idea for all people of all ages. Once the series of three oral vaccines is taken, however, there is no need for further boosters. So the only two things that an adult will wind up having to contend with are tuberculin tests and tetanus shots.

Tuberculin tests are generally administered by many physicians nowadays at the time of one's annual physical. A positive tuberculin test usually precludes any other tuberculin testing in the future and, in some cases, may actually result in the administration of certain medicines. This, of course, your doctor will decide with you. Negative tests, however, are usually repeated every year.

Some physicians give the tetanus-diphtheria toxoid, similar to what is given in children, to adults. Others feel that plain tetanus toxoid is all that is necessary. The frequency of tetanus boosters is something which has been changing over the past 10 years or so. They used to be given on a yearly basis. Reactions, as well as effective blood levels, dictated a change to every 5 years. Currently, it is recommended that a booster be given only every 10 years. If a person is exposed to a contaminated injury and his last booster was within the past 5 years, no booster is required. If it is more than 5 years ago, many physicians will give another booster for such an injury, even though the 10-year interval has not yet been reached.

INFLUENZA

Influenza, contrary to much popular belief, is not just any bad cold in the winter. A bad cold in the winter can be due to any one of a host of viruses—all of which can produce nasal congestion, sore throat, and cough. Influenza is caused by only the influenza viruses, of which there are fewer than five types.

Influenza, along with the vast majority of viruses, is not at all susceptible to antibiotics. What helps us successfully to combat the influenza virus is our underlying resistance and our immunity. No one, however, is naturally immune to influenza unless he has recently had the infection and, even then, that immunity is transient, being almost completely gone within a year of the illness. But there is one other way to enhance our immunity against influenza and that is by vaccination.

Some virus vaccines, such as the measles vaccine so widely being distributed to our children nowadays, confer lifelong immunity once adequate vaccination has been completed. Unfortunately the influenza virus does not belong to this category. There are two chief reasons for this: For one, immunity to the influenza virus just doesn't last as long as other viruses such as measles and chickenpox; for another (and this is very important), the influenza virus possesses the ability to change itself, which is one factor always lacking in those viruses that confer lifelong immunity.

During periods of epidemics, the causative factor is usually a new sub-variant of the influenza virus against which most people do not have protective levels of antibodies in their blood because of the very newness of this sub-variant. The natural ability of the virus to constantly change its internal pattern makes it unlikely that we will ever develop a permanent one-series type of vaccine against influenza.

In the 25 years since the introduction of the inactivated-virus influenza vaccines, there have been three major internal changes in the A-virus alone (the other major influenza virus is the B strain). The original A strain had so changed itself that, by 1947, the A-1 virus was essentially a new strain, and therefore practically no one had any immunity to it. This is what happened in the famous 1957 "Asian flu" epidemic. By that time the new virus was A-2, and again no one really had any immunity to it.

Influenza has generally not been an illness that hits a geographic area yearly; rather it tends to occur in a peak-wave every third to fifth year and then subsides for another 3 to 5 years.

Periodic vaccinations are recommended during epidemic years for most people (always excluding those people who are allergic to feathers, eggs, and other fowl products since the virus is grown in eggs and can cause a severe allergic reaction in these people). However, the influenza viruses don't disappear in the years between epidemics. They are constantly in the environmental background and can cause serious illness in persons who are unusually susceptible. There is a special group of people, such as people with chronic respiratory or cardiac disabilities—chronic bronchitis, emphysema, history of rheumatic fever with residual cardiac damage—for whom it is recommended that yearly vaccinations, even in nonepidemic years, be considered by their physicians. Most people over the age of 55 or 60 should also be considered for regular prophylactic injections against influenza. One class of persons for whom such recommendations are always in order, but who seem to be frequently forgotten, are pregnant women. The vaccines are killed-virus vaccines, containing no live virus, so that there is no danger of inadvertent infection of the mother or fetus. A report in the *New England Journal of Medicine* described the death of a mother and fetus because of influenza pneumonia in someone who had not had any protection for some years prior to this occurrence.

Influenza pneumonia, though, is an unusual complication of influenza. Generally, the condition is a mild one with some chills and fever, generalized aches and pains (most pronounced in the back and legs), headache, and weakness. Often there is a sore throat, a dry cough, and sometimes nasal congestion. While all these symptoms can cause discomfort, they are usually not serious. If the respiratory symptoms or increasing severity of cough or fever of over 101° persist for more than 5 days, then the rare but nonetheless serious complication of influenza pneumonia must be considered.

A new medication, amantadine, has been proposed as a preventive for certain forms of Type A influenza. Unfortunately, you have to take it by mouth twice a day for at least 10 days and sometimes up to 30 days; so the prevention may be worse than the disease. Generally, in an attack of acute uncomplicated influenza, bed rest for a day or so until the temperature has become normal is a good idea. A light diet with some extra fluids is also helpful. Aspirin is useful in lowering the temperature and relieving the discomfort of the muscle and back aches that the patients often experience.

INFECTIOUS MONONUCLEOSIS

The underlying mystery regarding a disease which, for many years, was listed in the medical textbooks as being of totally unknown cause may finally have bitten the dust. Infectious mononucleosis—so prevalent—so manifold in the degrees of the severity of its manifestations—was for so long so mysterious. Though it is not yet absolutely proven, there does seem very strong evidence that infectious mononucleosis is caused by a virus—the so-called Epstein-Barr virus. If this recent discovery turns out to be true, medicine will be faced once again with that peculiar occurrence of the same virus causing two very different diseases—one almost always benign, and the other one almost always very serious. This is, in a way, like the case of the same virus causing chickenpox in children and shingles in adults.

The disease we know as infectious mononucleosis is probably the same condition that was known as glandular fever years ago because the most typical "give away" symptom is the presence of rather significantly enlarged lymph glands in various parts of the body. It is a disease which is widespread throughout the world and occurs mainly between the ages of 15 and 30 years. For many years, the method of catching it was in doubt. Members of the same family rarely got it. Roommates didn't get it. Other people, however, who come in close contact with patients did seem to get it, and so the question of its transmission was a real problem. The current thinking is that this is probably not a virus which is carried freely through the air, such as cold viruses are. Rather it requires intimate contact with infected secretions for it to be transmitted. This is why for years it was also known as the "kissing disease." It seems that salivary contact between people does result in a highly effective way of transmitting the disease from one to the other and may very well be the chief way of catching the disease in most people.

The hallmark of infectious mononucleosis is lymph node enlargement, an enlargement which can occur in almost every lymph node in the body. Although the ones in the neck are often the most prominently involved, enlargement of the groin nodes or armpit nodes or even of those above the elbow or behind the ears is possible. As a matter of fact, there is good evidence that the deep internal lymph nodes of our body, which cannot be felt from the outside, may also become enlarged in the course of the disease. Medical pathologists often consider the spleen a form of large internal lymph node and indeed the spleen can become massively enlarged during the course of infectious mononucleosis. Where generally the disease has almost always been considered a benign condition, some have died from it. The few cases of people who have died have almost always been those patients who suffered a hemorrhagic rupture of the manifestly enlarged spleen from, for example, a blunt trauma or similar accident in most cases.

The second chief manifestation is the presence of fever. Usually the disease will have an incubation period of a month or so followed by the patient's developing vague "flulike" symptoms; he just doesn't feel well; he is tired; often he will have a headache and chilliness.

Sore throat is quite common and at times has been confused with strep throat because the inflamed throat will often be associated with enlargement of tonsilar tissue (if it's still there) and the presence of a whitish exudate that can look like that which is found in strep throats. These are the symptoms that are found in almost everyone with mono. However, since virtually every organ of the body can be involved, one individual case may differ from another one. Thus a person may have stiff neck, severe headache, tenderness of the eye-balls, etc., all of which could indicate irritation of the lining of the brain and spinal cord by the infection. Others who have the rare lung involvement will have shortness of breath, cough, and even some chest pain. Not infrequently, a fading, raised, slightly rose-red rash may be seen during some time in the course of the condition.

The diagnosis of the disease is no longer very difficult to arrive at, now that there are new sophisticated blood tests that can relatively quickly point out to the examining physician the presence of the special antibodies that are always present in cases of people with infectious mononucleosis. Further, a blood test (the white blood count) also will show the presence of unusually shaped white blood cells which are virtually diagnostic of the condition.

Most cases usually clear up within 3 weeks, although it is not unusual for it to last as long as 2 or 3 months. Complete cure is almost inevitable, although a strong folklore has built up regarding the possibility of relapses from mono. Though they occur much less frequently than people boast of having them, nonetheless relapses are possible; and most physicians are still not too sure whether the relapse occurred because the patient was allowed to be up and about too soon or whether it would have occurred regardless of what the patient did.

The treatment for "mono" is fairly standard nowadays. Since it is caused by a virus infection, antibiotics have no role in this condition. As a matter of fact, since a virus is the cause, there is no specific remedy for "mono." Usually, the physician takes the cue from the patient himself regarding treatment suggestions. Bed rest is always a good idea during the acute phase, and the patient is usually so weak and tired that he is more than happy to accede to the physician's orders. Another good reason for the bed rest is that sometimes the liver is inflamed and enlarged in "mono," and bed rest is very salutary for almost all conditions of inflamed or enlarged liver, regardless of the cause. Fluids should be taken freely. Patients whose temperature becomes very high (usually over 103 degrees), may take aspirin on a regular basis to help bring the temperature down towards a more normal range. The use of cortisone compounds is rarely, if ever, indicated in infectious mononucleosis.

It was stated at the beginning of the article that it would be very interesting indeed if it is proved that the Epstein-Barr virus is responsible for infectious mononucleosis. For a number of years now, the Epstein-Barr virus has been accepted as the proven cause for a very rare disease called Burkitt's Lymphoma. This disease, which was originally discovered in Africa and still is found almost exclusively in that continent, is a potentially fatal type of cancer of the lymph nodes. The lymph nodes are more massively involved than in cases of mononucleosis but, in a number of respects, the early stages of the diseases can be confused with each other. If it turns out that they are both caused by one single virus, then one of the most fascinating mysteries of the 20th century faces us: Why, in one part of the world, does the virus make youngsters sick and then allows almost all of them to recover, and in another part of the world it causes such severe cancerous change in the body that about 50% of the afflicted die from it?

Finally, for those of you who are worried, there has never been any evidence that mononucleosis has ever led to Burkitt's Lymphoma. They are really two separate diseases.

DISEASES FROM PETS

A recent estimate by the American Humane Society put the number of cats and dogs in American households as pets at about 70 million. While it is undoubtedly true that the overwhelming majority of such pets are completely safe from the point of view of transmitting infections to their human masters, it is equally true that there *are* diseases that can be acquired from them. This brief view of such infections will only cover the most common or the most serious of them.

Perhaps the most dreaded infectious disease in the world is rabies. This is, primarily, a virus disease of animals which attacks humans only after such animal exposure as a bite from a rabid animal or getting the saliva of such an animal onto a cut in the skin. The chief culprit, over the years, in infecting people has been the dog, but with the intensive vaccination of dogs against this over the past 15 to 25 years, it is becoming a less frequent cause, giving way instead to wild animals. There is a constant, large reservoir of the virus in many wild animals, especially the skunk, fox, wolf, coyote, squirrel, and raccoon. Not only can these animals transmit the infection directly to humans, but they serve as a pool from which dog infections continually arise. The disease, once acquired, is almost uniformly fatal not only in humans but also in the animals from which they caught it—with one serious exception. Bats seem to be able to harbor the rabies virus without getting sick from it all—and can continually infect dogs or humans.

Another infection humans usually acquire from dogs is leptospirosis. While this is a relatively uncommon condition, it can be quite serious and even fatal. Among the manifestations of the disease are fever, chills, conjunctivitis, severe muscle aches, rash, meningitis, kidney damage, and, less commonly, jaundice. The most common way humans catch the disease is through contact with water which is contaminated with the urine of dogs who are infected with the disease. Of course direct contact with contaminated dog urine is also a factor in infection. Usually the infection enters through a cut in the skin, but it can also enter via the mucous membranes of the nose, the mouth, or the eye.

One of the chief reasons dogs and cats should be dewormed regularly is to prevent their transmitting the disease known as visceral larva migrans. This usually mild condition (which can last 6–18 months, however) can be associated with fever, bronchitis, enlarged liver and spleen, and sometimes even a form of pneumonia. It is a disease especially common in children because uncovered sandboxes often turn out to be the culprit. Infected dogs and cats find them attractive places for defecation. The parasites eggs can then easily be transferred directly to the mouth as the child plays in contaminated soil.

Another disease transmitted by exposure to contaminated dog or cat feces has a similar name: cutaneous larva migrans. It too can be prevented by regular deworming of pets. Again, the parasite is deposited on the ground in dog or cat feces and can thrive in warm moist ground or sand. (That is why such infections seem to be especially common in seashore areas.) This time, however, the larva gets in through the intact, exposed skin usually on the feet, legs, or buttocks. The parasite then tunnels under the superficial layers of the skin leaving a winding, threadlike trail of inflammation and fluid-filled blisters which can easily become infected. Itching is quite common.

Another infection we can often get from cats and dogs is a bacterial infection which can follow a bite by one of them. There isn't too much we can do to prevent it in the way of pretreatment of cats and dogs. About 50% of such healthy pets carry the organisms, and the only thing one can do is to avoid getting bitten. An infected bite will usually manifest itself a few hours after the occurrence with localized redness, swelling, pain, and tenderness. This can often progress to a localized abscess at the site of the bite and also up at the lymph node region which drains the involved area. Antibiotics are required for cure.

Two recently widely publicized diseases that we can catch from cats are cat scratch fever and toxoplasmosis. Although the former usually does follow a scratch, it can also be subsequent to a cat bite, usually from a healthy animal. It begins as a tender pimple which soon becomes a scab-covered blister. Once again the draining lymph nodes enlarge and may become abscessed. Usually the entire condition clears up without any treatment.

Toxoplasmosis has received publicity lately not so much for the sickness it causes in those primarily infected as for the damage to the unborn child that can occur, especially if the woman infected is in the last trimester of her pregnancy when she contracts the infection. There are a number of ways this infection can be caught: from eating undercooked meat from an infected animal (*e.g.,* raw or poorly-cooked hamburger) or from contact with infected cats or their feces. The disease itself is very mild, usually manifesting itself as a few days of fever and lymph node enlargement. It's probably because of the very mildness and nonspecific nature of the symptoms that the condition is rarely specifically diagnosed. Yet, surprisingly, about a third of all adults in the U.S. give evidence in their blood of immunity to the disease, meaning that, knowingly or not, they must have had it sometime in the past.

Another disease from pets that has recently received much publicity is salmonellosis from pet baby turtles. Salmonellosis is a form of gastroenteritis with abdominal discomfort and diarrhea usually being the main symptoms, presenting themselves 12–48 hours after exposure. Exposure usually occurs when children handle pet turtles and put their fingers in their mouths, when turtle water is dumped into the kitchen sink, or when turtles are placed in dishes used for food.

Then there are those diseases which birds can transmit directly to humans, the most well known of which is psittacosis. This is really a disease of parakeets, which is usually acquired by man from the inhalation of dried bird excreta or from handling infected birds. Psittacosis can be manifested by fever, headache, and a pneumonialike infiltration of the lungs.

A fancy disease from birds is bird fancier's lung which is an allergic pneumonialike reaction with chills, fever, shortness of breath, and cough. Usually the attacks are of an allergic nature and occur within a few hours of handling birds.

SINUSITIS

Sometimes the holes in our head can cause us a lot of trouble. The subject of this article is that set of inner holes in our skulls that are called the paranasal sinuses. No one really knows, however, what is the chief purpose of having these "Swiss cheese" holes in the skull. Some people think that they are a concomitant to the evolutionary increase in brain size in higher animals; that is, the bigger the brain, the larger the hard bony skull needed to surround and protect it. Bone, however, is extremely heavy; and it is postulated that the presence of these openings scattered throughout the front half of the skull serves to lighten the bone load significantly.

Another theory is that the lining of the sinuses serves as a very efficient producer of antibodies that would help fight off or cure upper respiratory infections. The offending bacteria or viruses, by landing in the paranasal sinuses on their way from the nose down to the throat and lungs, cause enough of a reaction in these sinuses to help trigger the body's protective antibody mechanism. And that is really what this article is about—sinus infections.

There are four sets of these cavities in the normal skull. The largest are the maxillary sinuses which lie directly beneath the cheek bones on both sides. The frontal sinuses lie above the eyebrows and are actually joined in the midline. The ethmoid sinuses lie deeper in the skull immediately behind the upper part of the bridge of the nose, and the sphenoid sinuses are even further behind them in the central part of the skull cavity.

Each sinus is filled with air and has a small opening that leads out of it and connects to the upper inside part of the nose. This air passage is critically important, for if the sinuses were merely air-filled sacs with no outside connections, the air would painfully try to expand when we went to low-outside pressure areas and would equally painfully try to contract in high-pressure areas. If there were no passage to allow for these pressure equalizations, then we would really have cause to complain of sinus headaches! As a matter of fact, most sinus headaches are due to temporary blockage by mucus or growths of just these outlet-equalization-passages.

The mucous membrane lining of each of the eight sinuses is the same type of, and is actually in continuity with, the mucous membranes of the nose. Therefore, everything that can happen to the latter can happen to the former: irritation, congestion, mucus flow, etc.

What are some of the factors that can lead to or at least predispose one to a sinus attack? Many, among which some of the most common ones are:

1. Inadequate drainage due to a passage blockage which we mentioned above. This can be caused by a deviated nasal septum or polyps, etc.
2. Chronic infection and inflammation of the nose.
3. General weakened condition, such as after a serious illness.
4. Exposure to varying extremes in temperature or humidity, or both.
5. Emotional upset.
6. Dental abscess, which can cause a maxillary sinusitis because the maxillary sinus sits right on top of the upper teeth.
7. Allergy
8. Tobacco smoke or other heavy pollutants.

There are other predisposing factors, but these are among the most important.

Sinus conditions can be considered either acute or chronic. Acute sinusitis may be either sudden or gradual in onset and generally occurs in the course of a head cold. Headache, nasal and postnasal discharge, pain over the involved sinuses, and a general feeling of being ill are among the most prominent symptoms. Some people may have fever of 2 or even 3 degrees, some may lose their sense of smell temporarily, others may have a toothache, especially if the maxillary sinuses are involved, and still others may experience a somewhat rare swelling around the eyes. If one presses hard over the affected sinus, the patient usually experiences pain.

The picture of chronic sinusitis is much less dramatic than most of the above symptoms. Perhaps the one symptom that is almost always present is headache, and often the location of the headache helps pinpoint which of the four sets of sinuses is involved. Thus, pain over the forehead and around the eyes usually means involvement of the frontal sinuses. Pain over the upper teeth or in the cheek below the eyes usually is maxillary sinus involvement. Since the sphenoid and ethmoid sinuses are much deeper in the head, the pain they cause can be referred to almost any part of the skull. Thus, pain in the back of the head is often caused by sphenoid sinus involvement, even though the sphenoid sinus itself is in the front half of the skull. The involvement of these two sets of sinuses can also cause pain behind the root of the nose, behind the eyes, and even in the neck.

In sinus inflammation not only is the nasal mucosa swollen and red but very often there is the presence of thick, yellowish green mucus, and this is the dividing line used by many physicians in determining how they will treat sinus infections. A viral sinus infection usually has little, if any, fever and the mucus remains clear and whitish even though all the other symptoms of pain and discomfort are just as present as if it were a bacterial infection. However, when a bacterial sinusitis supervenes, then a person's temperature usually rises, only rarely above 102 or so, and the discharge may become thick, yellow, and even greenish. The latter type of involvement calls for the administration of an antibiotic. There are a number of antibiotics that are recommended; but penicillin, tetracycline, and erythromycin are the three chief effective antibiotics for bacterial sinus infections. When there is no evidence of bacterial involvement, judicious, restricted use of vasoconstrictors may be given to the patient. These may be given either in the form of nose drops, which the patient usually has to apply when he is lying down with the head bent over backwards, in the form of commercial nasal sprays, or even in the form of decongestants taken by mouth. All can be effective in achieving the primary purpose of the use of decongestants, which is to permit adequate drainage and ventilation of the involved sinuses. However, if such decongestants are used more than three or four times a day, a pernicious condition called reactive hyperemia can result, which is almost worse than the original condition itself. What happens is the decongestant causes the mucus membrane blood vessels to constrict, the swelling diminishes, and the air passage is clear. However, when the medication wears off, the blood vessels become very wide open and there is a rebound congestion. The person then uses more decongestant to try to get those blood vessels to go back into spasm and clear the air passages. This may work once or twice, but it is of the order of whipping a tired horse. After a while those blood vessels are unable to react to any medication and remain dilated and fixed in the wide open position, causing massive blockage and congestion of the nasal passages. The aim of decongestant therapy should be to give three or four 2–3 hour periods a day of nasal decongestion to help drain the involved areas without the futile expectation of having clear nasal passages throughout the whole day.

Chronic sinusitis, if due to allergy, will possibly respond to desensitization; if due to nasal obstruction, reparative surgery may be occasionally required. A person with chronic sinusitis should be instructed in the proper manner of blowing his nose and also cautioned against blowing it too often or too vigorously. The nose should be blown with the mouth open, one nostril at a time.

Warm saline lavages are often helpful in clearing the clogged material in both acute and chronic sinusitis and are always a good adjunct to whatever form of therapy is used.

STUFFY NOSE

Probably one of the most frequent of all medical complaints is a stuffy nose—and its causes are many and varied indeed, ranging all the way from a mild cold to, on rare occasions, a malignant tumor.

A first approach to the problem is to find out how long the patient has had the symptoms. If only for a few days, then one must consider the possibility of an acute infection—either bacterial or viral in origin. The overwhelming majority of such "stuffy noses of brief duration" are due to the common cold—which actually can be caused by any of a host of viruses. One hallmark that is quite reliable in differentiating a viral from a bacterial nasal infection is the quality of the mucous discharge. A thick yellowish discharge is probably due to a bacterial infection—either one that was bacterial from the beginning or that was a viral infection that became "superinfected" by a bacterium. While antibiotics are of absolutely no value in virus colds, their use should be *considered* (but this does not necessarily mean that they should always be *used*) in bacterial infections.

If there is a headache accompanying the "stuffy nose of brief duration," the possiblity that the infection has traveled up into the sinuses should be considered. The above antibiotic suggestions also hold for an acute sinusitis.

One final possibility to consider with regard to young children is the possibility that the child has pushed a foreign body up his nostril which, of course, would have to be removed before the condition will clear up.

Now we turn to those causes of stuffy nose that are truly of chronic duration (weeks to months, even to years). A first approach to these might be to determine if the blockage is on one or both sides. A very common cause for unilateral blockage of long standing is the impaired drainage secondary to a deviated septum, either from a previous injury or, in some cases, having been that way from birth. In some cases of badly deviated septa, surgery has offered excellent relief.

When a unilateral blockage is associated with unusual sneezing accompanied by a loss of the sense of smell, the possiblity of a polyp (which is an almost-always benign overgrowth of inner nasal structure tissue) must be considered. However, if these symptoms are associated with pain, bleeding, and a foul odor (detectable by others), the possiblity of an internal malignant tumor must be considered and other extensive studies must be performed to prove or disprove this. Incidentally, a benign polyp usually responds quite satisfactory to removal by surgery.

When one is dealing with chronic nasal stuffiness that is *not* unilateral, one has to consider the possiblity of enlarged adenoids, especially in a child who is a chronic mouth breather and who has recurrent attacks of middle ear infections. Most children by the age of 5 have experienced significant shrinkage of tonsilar and adenoidal tissue that the chronic nasal stuffiness and mouth breathing should have subsided. If it hasn't, then surgical removal should be considered.

When there is a history of chronic nasal congestion with a history of bilateral or alternating blockage associated with loss of the sense of smell and a peculiar nasal twang to the voice, one has to consider the overuse of medical nasal decongestants, of either the spray or nose drop type.

If the chronic stuffy nose is associated with bilateral or alternating blockage, symptoms of watery, itchy eyes, nasal itchiness, and a seasonal type of nasal drip, the possiblity of a nasal allergy must be strongly considered. Often, in such cases, one will find a family history of allergy or even a personal history of allergies such as hives, eczema, asthma, or allergic conjunctivitis. When a doctor examines the mucous membrane or inner nasal lining in cases of nasal allergy, he often will find that lining pale and boggy, producing a clear, watery discharge. An examination of a smear of the nasal secretions will often result in the finding of a high percentage of specific "allergy cells" from the blood's white blood cell system. The finding of an excess of such cells usually will clinch the diagnosis of allergy. The treatment of such an allergic rhinitis includes the avoidance of the allergen (if it can be determined), possibly the use of specific desenitization injections conducted by an allergist, and even antihistamines, whose use, I hope you will have noticed, I have carefully avoided recommending until we reached this condition of true allergy.

There is one final condition to be considered in cases of chronic nasal congestion with a history of bilateral or alternating blockage—vasomotor rhinitis. Patients with this condition do not have the watery, itchy eyes or nose or seasonal nasal drip; rather, their symptoms are perennial but *do* worsen during temperature or humidity changes, and also during times when they are fatigued or emotionally upset. They will have only minimal nasal discharge, but there will be some postnasal drip. The cause of vasomotor rhinitis is not at all clear-cut. Many doctors suspect allergy, but these patients often do not have an allergic history. Some doctors who refer to this as an "oversensitive nose" suggest symptomatic treatment, by avoiding or at least trying to diminish the effect of those agents or causes which are most offending.

STREP THROAT

One important and common upper airways infection for which antibiotics are mandatory is the condition referred to as strep throat. Strep throats are caused by the streptococcus bacterium, are bacterial infections, and, therefore, are susceptible to antibiotics. Luckily for almost everyone concerned, the antibiotic most successfully used in the treatment and cure of strep throat is one of the mildest and best of them all: penicillin.

How does one distinguish the common cold from strep throat? The only definitive answer is by a throat culture which, nowadays, is much more easily obtained and relatively inexpensive than it was 20 or so years ago.

While a throat culture may give a definite answer, does that mean that every person with a sore throat should have a throat culture? The answer is "no." For, contrary to popular belief, the symptoms of a strep throat are usually not like those of a cold at all. It is quite common during the course of a common cold to develop a cough. A cough accompaning a strep throat is so rare that its presence is enough to make one wonder whether this is a strep throat in the first place. A common cold is invariably accompanied by a profuse, usually watery, mucous discharge from the nostrils. This symptom, more than anything else, is the hallmark in most people's minds of the common cold—and right they are. Strep throats, on the other hand, simply don't have this symptom. The presence of nasal discharge makes the condition much more likely to be a common cold than a strep throat.

Common colds do often have raspy throats. There is a burning irritation present in the back of the throat in many common colds, but usually the patient will not complain of severe pain on swallowing. Patients with strep throat indeed invariably have a "bad throat" with a *lot* of pain on swallowing. Not at all unusual in a common cold is involvement of the larynx with laryngitis, which is really another name for hoarseness of the voice due to inflamed swelling of the vocal cords. Laryngitis with voice changes is extremely unusual in strep throats. Sometimes the patient will whisper rather than speak with a strep throat because of the severe pain that even speaking causes him; but if he could bring himself to speak, one hears that he speaks in a normal voice and that he is not hoarse.

The common cold is often accompanied by malaise or some non-specific feeling of non-well-being. One feels unwell and perhaps even feverish although, not infrequently, the thermometer indicates that very slight temperature, if any, is present. Thus, a common cold rarely will have temperature of over 101 degrees. A strep throat, on the other hand, usually makes one much sicker. This is especially so in children. With a strep throat, one feels quite ill, weak, exhausted, and tired. The patient often will complain of a significant headache. The feeling of feverishness is often borne out by the presence of temperature, even in adults, of over 101 degrees.

Examination by a physician will reveal, in the common cold, a red throat; but usually there is little, if any, swelling of the throat tissues. In a strep throat the throat tissues are not only red but quite swollen. The tonsils, if still present, can become so enlarged that they almost close off the air passages. It is quite unusual in a common cold to have pus in the throat area; it is quite unusual in strep throat *not* to have pus in the throat area. In the common cold, the lymph nodes in the neck will be slightly enlarged, if at all; in strep throat, the lymph nodes are commonly quite enlarged, so much so that they become tender and painful. If your doctor does a blood count, he will usually find a normal blood count in a common cold and "a high white count" in strep throat.

As one can see, it almost seems there would be no way to confuse a common cold with a strep throat, but that is not correct. A mild strep throat or a very severe common cold can often mimic each other and so, again, it must be emphasized that the only way the diagnosis can be made definitively is by a throat culture.

Some physicians, knowing about the potentially serious complications of strep infections, will take a throat culture and send it to the laboratory; but they treat the patient immediately with antibiotics before the culture results are known. This practice is not necessarily a bad one, except that it may expose the patient to potentially sensitizing antibiotics unnecessarily if it turns out that he has a negative throat culture. Many laboratories can get the result of a throat culture back to the doctor within 1 or 2 days, and it has been shown that the initiation of antibiotics 1 or 2 days, or even 3 or 4 days, after the onset of the strep throat is satisfactory, if given long enough, to prevent the complications of strep infections.

Two questions remain: How long should treatment be given?

What complications? For very complex medical reasons, some of which we know and some of which we have no idea about, it is imperative that antibiotics be given in strep throats for a full 10 days. Penicillin is the antibiotic of choice but, if the person is allergic to penicillin, erythromycin is a good alternative. Regardless of how well the patient may feel after 1 or 2 days of antibiotics, they should not be discontinued until the full 10 days have gone by.

What complications? Rheumatic fever and acute glomerulonephritis or "Bright desease," as it is also called, can occur. While many a person can go through a strep throat unscathed and not develop these two, late, noninfectious complications of the strep throat, others *will* get them; and since there is no way of telling in advance, the best medical therapy is to treat everyone who has a diagnosed strep throat.

RHEUMATIC FEVER AND NEPHRITIS

In the preceding article, we discussed acute streptococcal infections, especially strep throats, which are their most common manifestation. The importance of 10 days' duration of antibiotics for all such infections was stressed, not so much because you need 10 days worth of medications to control the strep infection (antibiotics usually do a very satisfactory job on strep throats in 3 to 5 days), but because it was learned about 20 to 30 years ago that prolonged treatment for strep infections was a major factor in reducing the occurrence of acute rheumatic fever and acute glomerulonephritis (Bright's disease). These two conditions had been for centuries among the most debilitating and serious of the life-threatening chronic diseases of mankind.

While the picture is far from clear scientifically as to just what is going on to cause these diseases, an oversimplification, nonetheless, is helpful. It seems as if there are parts of the streptococcus organism that for some peculiar reason resemble certain chemical components of human heart and human kidney. When a strep infection is added to this background fact, a funny thing occurs. While it is true that, in the days before antibiotics, some people literally died of strep infections, recovery was the rule and not the exception. How did people recover? By building up antibodies in their own blood stream specifically directed against the antigenic components of the streptococcus bacteria. The formation of these antibodies would be triggered by the presence of the strep infection. Once triggered, these antibodies would be produced in massive quantities, would rush through the blood stream to the involved infected parts of the body, and there would combine with, neutralize, and efficiently kill the particular organism against which they had been formed. Fortunately, there would be enough antibody kill of the infected organisms that the person would get over his infection without the aid of antibiotics. This was all fine as far as the strep infection itself went, but something peculiar was happening in some people, and that was, simplistically stated, something like this: Once triggered, in these people (and there was and still is no way of telling who these people are beforehand), the antibody production mechanism would not shut off, even though it had succeeded in neutralizing and destroying all the infecting organisms. As a result, one had millions and billions of antibody molecules floating throughout the blood stream but no bacterial antigen to combine with them. These antibody molecules were, in other words, like "an accident looking for a place to happen." What did happen is that they would often combine with whatever chemical parts of tissues that resembled the organisms which had triggered their production in the first place. As a result, these antibodies were combined with human heart muscle and human kidney tissue because these were the parts that chemically were similar to the strep organisms. This inadvertent chemical reaction caused severe inflammation of the combining parts with resulting swelling, tissue disruptions, ingress of reparative cells from the blood stream, etc. This whole undesirable reaction resulted in the two diseases above mentioned. When it afflicted the heart and the joints, the disease was called acute rheumatic fever; when it afflicted the kidneys, it was called acute glomerulonephritis (Bright's disease). There is even a minority of "these high antibody reactors" in whom the combining tissue was not the heart, not the joints, not the kidneys, but the brain itself, and the condition known as chorea or St. Vitus' dance resulted.

Acute rheumatic fever is called rheumatic because it usually is associated with joint swelling and pains. Its onset usually occurs well after the strep throat has subsided, often 3 or 4 weeks later. It is as if as long as there were bacteria around to absorb the antibodies nothing bad was happening. Once the bacteria were gone, then the antibody buildup had to reach a certain critical point before damage could occur. Luckily, these migrating joint symptoms of pain and swelling, while uncomfortable and in many cases temporarily incapacitating, did not result in any permanent joint damage. On the other hand, the swelling and ingress into body tissues of cells that occurs during the infection and healing of the heart involvement, does result in permanent damage, especially to one or more of the heart's four valves. Often there is such severe scarring that the valve no longer functions correctly, becomes leaky, and the long-term consequence is chronic severe heart valve damage, often terminating in premature death. Once a person has had rheumatic fever, he is more likely to have a second attack than someone who has not had it before, and each attack leaves more damage. Strep throats should be treated vigorously in everyone but especially in people who have ever had one attack of rheumatic fever, to try to prevent further damage. Unfortunately, since rheumatic fever is not an infection in itself, it doesn't respond to antibiotics—rather, if the attack is brought to the physician's attention early enough, it can be more or less controlled by massive doses of aspirin and various cortisone compounds. But the crux of the matter in rheumatic fever is not the always unsatisfactory partial treatment of the condition, but rather the often completely satisfactory prevention of the condition by vigorous treatment of all strep infections.

Acute glomerulonephritis involves swelling and distortion of various structures in the kidneys with resultant loss of some kidney functions. The kidneys tend to keep important blood proteins from being lost in the urine. In nephritis, that function is often lost. The filtering function of the kidneys is their prime function, and this is often affected also so that the person will not only have swelling of the body because of accumulation of fluids but also the retention of various toxic metabolic products in his blood stream, which can cause severe mental dulling and debility. Often there is marked high blood pressure because of the kidney's role in blood pressure control is affected. Again, there is no treatment for nephritis, just various forms of palliation. The watchword is once more "prevention."

What is the role of prolonged antibiotic treatment in prevention? Well, we are not at all sure of the complete role. Nonetheless, we know it is something like this: If a person receives antibiotics to wipe out the bacteria, there is no need for his body to keep making antibodies. As a matter of fact, if the antibiotics are administered early enough, the person's antibody triggering mechanism will never be triggered. As a result, the dangerous output of excessive antibodies will be nipped, so to speak, in the bud. There is one theory that holds that even though the major symptoms of the strep throat have gone, there remain pockets of asymptomatic strep bacteria in the body which prolong the excessive antibody production. This makes a lot of sense because it is well known that, even if you treat a strep infection late, even a week or so late (when presumably most people's antibody mechanisms have been triggered), the incidence of rheumatic fever and nephritis is markedly diminished.

TETANUS

One of the most dreaded of all diseases that can afflict mankind is tetanus, or lockjaw as it is commonly called. It is a disease which could affect anyone, regardless of age. It is one in which the main medical thrust is toward prevention because treatment of the condition is very uncertain and, unfortunately, often unsuccessful. Last year alone, it has been estimated that there were about 350,000 cases of tetanus worldwide, almost half of which resulted in death.

Tetanus is a bacterial disease. The usual course is a break in the intactness of the human skin. Such a wound does not always have to be a serious injury since even trivial injuries have allowed introduction of tetanus spores under the skin.

One of the chief causes of wound contamination is such an item as soil (especially if it is contaminated with human or animal feces)— which makes the disease especially common among agricultural workers.

Tetanus differs from other bacterial infections in that the local problem may be minimal while the systemic problems are what cause death. The reason for this is that the tetanus bacteria make a deadly nerve poison which is absorbed into the blood stream and circulates throughout the body. Thus, the local wound, while it may look infected, often does not look much worse than any other localized skin infection, even though the patient at the time may be dying from the nerve poison that is being elaborated by the wound bacteria.

There are varying degrees of tetanus, the milder the better. One fairly reliable indicator is the length of time elapsed between the con-tamination incident and the onset of the tetanus itself. If more than 9 days have gone by, the patient will usually not have a severe attack. Usually, the mild attacks have stiffness of the muscles; sometimes this rigidity is severe enough to cause pain. Often only one limb is affected in mild cases. The classical "lockjaw" is caused by stiffness of the jaw muscles themselves.

The more severe case of tetanus usually has generalized stiffness of the whole body, and the locking jaw is so spastic that the mouth can hardly be opened. A characteristic leer is sometimes present because of the spasm of the entire set of facial muscles. Sometimes, the pa-tient with moderately severe tetanus will have some mild difficulty in swallowing which will make him cough or splutter while drinking—caused by spasm of the throat muscles. It is this which leads to one of the frequent secondary complications of tetanus: pneumonia, caused by food or liquids going into the lungs since they had slipped into the windpipe instead of the gullet while being swallowed.

The truly severe cases of tetanus have all of the above symptoms plus massive muscle spasms, often causing the body to arch back as if the head were trying to touch the heels. The strength of these spasms may be so intense that they may result in spinal backbone fractures. Sometimes there is so much spasm of the breathing mus-cles that the patient becomes bluish from lack of air. He could de-velop fever and profuse sweating, the heart could race, often in an erratic rhythm, and the blood pressure could go sky-high.

In short, tetanus is one disease that would be nice never to get. Once it has set in, sedatives and tranquilizers are used to help control the muscle spasm. The original wound must be laid wide open so that much air can get to it. This tends to prevent further multiplication of the bacteria and thus would diminish their elaboration of the nerve poison. High doses of penicillin help to kill the bacteria, but they do not neutralize the nerve poison that has already been produced. What is needed for that is tetanus antitoxin. Up until very recently, this antitoxin was a horse serum product; and we had to keep our fingers crossed in the hope that the patient would not manifest a seri-ous reaction to the horse serum. In recent years, however, there is a human tetanus immune globulin available which causes many fewer, if any, of the allergic type reactions that were being seen with the horse serum.

If the above listed items make the cure sound almost worse than the disease, there is something to that. What then should be done about the tetanus problem? Luckily there is an answer, and it's a marvelous one if only people would take advantage of it. The answer lies in the realm of prevention and is called active immunization against tetanus.

All children should receive DPT shots (diphtheria-pertussis-tetanus). The first one is usually given in the first 6 months or so after birth. A booster then follows at approximately 18 months of age, and a final booster is given shortly before the child enters school. For adults who have never received the childhood immunization, the recommendation is: two shots at least 4 weeks apart, followed by a reinforcing injection 8–10 months later.

Once this basic series of injections has been completed, all that is needed is a booster injection every 10 years, which this will absolutely protect a person from the dreaded disease described above. The frequency of the booster shots has been the subject of recent medical research. Ten years or so ago it was felt that a person should receive a tetanus booster about every year. Studies then revealed that the booster was not necessary that often, and the recommendation was changed to every 5 years. The current reccomendations are for a booster shot every 10 years. Some of the new thinking (which some doctors may find a little too radical for their liking) says that if the booster shot was given within the past 5 years, another shot would not be required, even though the person has sustained a grossly contaminated injury. Other more traditional medical thinking would give a booster shot whenever such an injury occurs. In the absence of any severe injury, all that is required is a booster every 10 years. It does not sound like much, but it can prevent one of mankind's most dreaded disease.

Why not take a few minutes right now and check your records or your memory: Have you had a booster within the past 10 years?

TUBERCULOSIS

Tuberculosis is one of the oldest scourges of mankind. The "white death," as it was known in the Middle Ages, has been killing people for thousands of years; and even today, when so much progress has been made toward controlling it, tuberculosis is still a fearsome name.

As with most infectious diseases, tuberculosis plays no favorites. All humans are susceptible to it, and the best medical advice is not to get it in the first place. At one time, it was believed that the main ways of contracting it were via contaminated fingers, food, or eating utensils. While you *can* contract it in those ways, the chief way is via air-borne infection. Dr. Alexander Langmuir of the U.S. Public Health Service estimates that at least 95% of all tuberculosis in the United States is the result of air-borne infection.

There have been many approaches to the detection and treatment of TB, but in the past few years the entire approach has undergone a radical change—a reversal, in fact. A brief survey of previous approaches, however, can help us to understand some of the reasons behind the current medical stance.

Tuberculosis shares with syphilis the dubious honor not only of being one of mankind's greatest scourges, but also of not being caused by a very dangerously infective organism. Thus, if you get pneumonia or meningitis, within a week or two you either build up enough resistance to kill the bugs or they kill you, because such infections are caused by very virulent organisms. However, there are two organisms in man's environment that are of a relatively low virulence —those that cause TB and syphilis—and that's one of the main reasons they've been such persistent destroyers of man.

This seeming paradox can be partially explained by the concept of resistance to infection. Our body has a tremendous capacity to protect itself against the invasion of foreign matter. When a foreign particle such as a bacterium or a virus gets into our system and starts to multiply, it triggers our fixed antibody or our curculating antibody mechanisms. In a few days, we make so many millions of antibodies that they completely neutralize and overwhelm the invaders and we get well. Woe betide the person who's got something amiss with his antibody mechanism: the bug might win!

All of the above holds true for virulent organisms. The tuberculosis organism, however, is not very virulent. Primary tuberculosis, the name for the initial illness when one becomes infected with the bug, is not much of a sickness. It's not in the same league with such diseases as pneumonia, meningitis, or even strep throat. In essence, it does not present much of a threat to the body's defenses; and, as a result, it does not mobilize a dramatic antibody response. If it did, the bugs would be killed and that would be the end of it. Since it doesn't, the bugs don't all die but go underground in our bodies, so to speak. There they can survive for 70–80 years, locked in but smoldering, ready to break out at any time, causing major or minor periods of illness and damage to virtually every organ in the body. For tuberculosis is not only a disease of the lungs but can, over the years, go to the bones, the kidneys, the lymph nodes, the brain, the liver, the glands—anywhere. It is one of the most wide-ranging, devastating diseases that man can have, and all because, in essence, the causative bacterium is not virulent enough to trigger a killing antibody protective reaction.

Let us return to that primary tuberculosis infection. It is usually a very mild illness, a cold, for instance, that lasted a week or two longer than usual, a week or two of "not feeling well," a cough that lasted an extra week or two, a couple of weeks of some feverish feelings that went away before you found out what was going on.

During this period your body's antibody mechanism (especially the so-called fixed tissue antibody mechanism) was being triggered, but not to a killing degree. As a result, the antibodies that were formed took effect and helped you combat and lock in the infecting organisms. Many of the organisms—but not all—died and you got well again, but with your live bacteria locked into a nest of scar tissue, waiting, waiting.

Most doctors would draw a distinction between tuberculous infection and tuberculous disease. What has just been described is primary tuberculous infection. Tuberculous disease is what happens when those locked-in organisms break out and spread the disease throughout the body. In the "old days" when people still went to sanatoriums for tuberculosis, it was invariably the reactivation case that had to go. Primary infections were generally so mild and cleared up so quickly that it was the rare person indeed who had to go to a TB sanatorium to recuperate.

As a matter of fact, there was a sort of special immunity that was conferred on a person who had previously suffered from a mild primary tuberculous infection: It kept him from getting reinfected from the outside regardless of how often he seemed to come in contact with new tuberculosis organisms. The continued presence of locked-in but live tuberculosis organisms somehow caused a low-grade persisting antibody response that protected the person against further reexposure infections.

Of course, he was not protected against the deadlier form of tuberculosis—the reactivation form. So long as those bugs were alive in his body, the possibility of a flare-up was always present. Thus, if his resistance was lowered from some chronic disease such as diabetes, or as a result of stomach ulcer operations, old age, emphysema, or a nontuberculous pneumonia that was right near the scar focus with the live TB bugs, the bugs would break out and could spread all over, either directly or through the blood stream. Then, one had a full-fledged case of reactivation tuberculosis on one's hands. These people were sick, these people did need sanatoriums, they did die, often at tragically young ages.

It is a partially unexplainable fact that, in the United States at least, the prevalence of tuberculosis has been steadily decreasing since the turn of the century, long before the wonder-drug antibiotics against tuberculosis were introduced in the late 1940's. Maybe the decrease was due to better hygiene, maybe to better diet (with higher overall quantities of necessary proteins), maybe to factors we don't yet understand. The fact remains that tuberculosis is becoming rarer than ever in the United States.

In the early years of this century, when the likelihood of continual reexposure was high, the people who seemed best off, in the short run, were those who had overcome a primary infection. Although it made them liable to the long-term reactivation form if ever their resistance became critically low, it did afford them interim protection against reinfection, which was potentially a daily occurrence.

Now, how could one tell if he had had a primary tuberculosis infection? By a very simple test, the tuberculin skin test—also called a patch test, a Tine test, and other names, depending on the type and form of administration. Essentially, the test consisted of injecting into the skin either converted tuberculosis organisms or a purified protein derivative of those organisms. The body's antibody mechanism would recognize such an injection as being an "old friend" if a previous tuberculous infection had left behind some locked-in, live organism. Two or three days later, a small lump would appear at the site of injection. This would prove that the person was "tuberculin positive," meaning that at one time he had had a significant tuberculous infection (either the mild primary form or the more serious reactivation form).

Years ago, being tuberculin positive was a good thing. So great was its protection against frequent incidental reexposure that in the 1920's BCG was introduced for tuberculin-negative persons. BCG was a special bacillus which, when given to the person as a shot in the arm, would trigger the antibody mechanism against tuberculosis even though BCG was not the tuberculosis organism and even though it did not cause TB. What good was BCG? It made you tuberculin-test positive, which afforded protection against incidental exposures and primary tuberculous infections. And as an added bonus, since it really was not the tuberculosis organism, if your resistance ever did break down, you wouldn't come down with widespread tuberculosis since you never had true tuberculosis organisms in you to begin with. Yes, up until about 1960, it paid to be "positive."

All of that is changing rapidly. Not only is BCG not used anymore, but it no longer pays to be positive! What has happened? At least two things: (1) The amount of tuberculosis organisms in the natural environment has decreased, as we mentioned, and (2) the number of potential infectors (those having the organism) has diminished. This means that the likelihood of random exposure to TB has lessened. In short, the "negatives" are in less danger of contracting the disease.

Another major factor in our new feeling about the negatives has been the truly miraculous effect of the antituberculosis antibiotics—streptomycin, PAS, and isoniazid. TB can, in the overwhelming majority of cases, be arrested by these drugs. In fact, we can even speak of cures in some cases. Such persons are usually those who contracted their positivity within the preceding year or so. Because their bugs have not been locked in by too thick a wall of scar tissue, the drugs can still penetrate the scars and actually kill, for the first time, all the bugs. With the death of all the bugs, one reverts to tuberculin-negative. Then, no matter what happens to your resistance over the ensuing years, you're not likely to develop reactivation tuberculosis since you don't have any live TB organisms left in your system. And, as we said, primary infections are less likely because there are fewer TB organisms in the environment in the first place.

The new recommendations, then, are: Give children, parents—

everyone—a yearly tuberculin test. If they are negative, fine. Just keep checking them every year. Whenever they become positive, give them the drug treatment for TB—even though they feel well, even though they won't have to miss a day of work or school. They just take their medicines daily for a year or so and become tuberculin-negative again. Then, no matter what happens to their resistance, there will be no reactivations, no episodes of killer-tuberculosis, because they no longer have any live tuberculosis organisms left in their bodies. They are then retested each year and, along with anyone else who becomes positive, will be retreated for a year whenever necessary.

As you can see, the whole approach to the treatment of TB has been turned upside down, and it's one of the great pieces of news in man's fight against the killer disease—tuberculosis.

PARASITIC DISEASES

As travel increases in the summer, an increase is concomitantly noticed in intestinal parasitic infections among travelers. Since any organism which infects the gastrointestinal tract might be considered a parasite, it should be mentioned that that is not what is meant by a parasitic disease. When the infecting organism is either a virus or a bacterium, the resulting infection, though it may cause the sufferer lots of distress in the form of nausea, vomiting, and diarrhea, is nonetheless generally a self-limiting disease. Such an organism multiplies briefly in the human body, and then it and its toxic products are usually expelled within, at most, 2 weeks of the onset of the infection. Rarely indeed does any such organism actually invade and become a permanent dweller in the host's body.

Yet, that very last concept is what is meant, technically, by a parasitic disease. As such, it is quite evident that the great majority of travel-associated gastrointestinal afflictions are not of a parasitic nature. While they are rare, however, the fact that they can become indwellers in our body makes the conditions potentially far more serious than a run-of-the-mill virus or bacterial affliction.

One group of parasitic infections is that caused by the so-called roundworm. Among these infections, the most well known is probably hookworm infection. However, it, as well as most of the other roundworm infestations, is usually not caught through contaminated food, rather as a result of intimate exposure (such as walking barefoot) to contaminated soil. Ascariasis, however, is the one roundworm infection which *can* be contracted from eating contaminated food; in this case, vegetables. Though its distribution is worldwide, ascariasis is most common in warm, moist climates. During the early stages of infestation, pulmonary bronchial symptoms may predominate. Later, the symptoms are mainly in the gastrointestinal tract, often in the nature of colicky pains. Rarely the patient may pass a true worm either by vomiting or in the stool. While this is the most visibly dramatic of all the parasitic infestations, it is not the most serious since medicine is available to rid one of the condition.

The second major class of parasitic infestations includes the tapeworms, chief among which are the beef, pork, and fish tapeworm. While the beef and fish tapeworms are probably of worldwide distribution, the pork tapeworm is more common in Latin American, Asia, Russia, and Eastern Europe. Not only can tapeworm infections cause gastronintestinal symptoms, but they can also make a person systemically ill. The fish tapeworm can even cause anemia. Again, as is the case with just about all the parasitic infestations, medicines are available for their successful eradication. Of course, prophylaxis is the ideal approach; and that involves thorough cooking of suspected beef, of pork in infected areas, and thoroughly cooking or freezing fresh-water fish.

The third class of intestinal parasites is that class called the protozoa. The chief representatives are amebiasis and giardiasis. Amebiasis is one of the most serious of all the parasitic infestations and may even be the most common one. Amebiasis occurs worldwide and can be contracted from contaminated water or food. It can be a treacherous infestation in that the gastrointestinal symptoms may be quite limited in many people even though the classical picture ("amebic dysentery") is more severe. The serious consequence of amebiasis is that this parasite can go to the liver and can cause amebic hepatitis and even liver abscesses. There are medicines available to eradicate it depending on what organ system is involved, but the medicine in some instances is potentially toxic.

While giardiasis was once thought not worth treating, many people get enough diarrhea, abdominal pain, and even some weight loss that the current recommendation is that it be treated. Luckily, the treatment is relatively easy and quite effective.

The final class of intestinal parasites are the flukes: intestinal, liver, lung, or blood. While all of these are rare in the United States, they are very prevalent, especially in the Orient and in tropical countries as well as Africa and Latin America. The blood fluke causes schistosomiasis. Were it not for the fact that most cases of schistosomiasis are concentrated in pockets of the Far East and the Near East, it would surely rank above amebiasis as the most serious of the worldwide parasitic infestations. The various fluke infestations are contracted by eating contaminated foods: the intestinal fluke by contaminated vegetables, fresh-water fish, and snails; the liver fluke by eating contaminated watercress or fresh-water fish; the lung fluke by crabs or crayfish; the blood fluke usually by being exposed to snail infested water (even swimming in such water can result in its entry through the intact skin). The chief area of symptoms is revealed by the specific name of the fluke involved. While treatment exists for the various fluke infestations, the course of treatment is complex, and some of the medicines used can be quite toxic.

11
cMetabolic

DIABETES

There was a time when being afflicted with diabetes was something people tried to keep secret. If there was a history of diabetes in the family, it too was treated as a deep, dark secret for fear that if the word got out, no one would marry your sisters.

Things have changed—somewhat. The stigma of having diabetes personally is essentially gone. Diabetics, even severe ones if under good treatment, socialize, marry, even have children (a risky business in the old preinsulin days, when the basic disease often resulted in a significant decrease in the ability to get pregnant and, in those cases in which pregnancy did occur, the situation was often fraught with grave danger both to the mother and the developing child), and hold down responsible jobs in all strata of American life. The old fear about keeping a family history of diabetes secret was, however, based on what may very well be one of the basic truths of diabetes: The tendency towards the disease is strongly hereditary; and, while the days of secrecy and shame are luckily long since past, nonetheless, to deny or make little of this hereditary tendency is not only inaccurate but could be dangerous. For those who have inherited a tendency towards the disease, far better to know of it, and to keep an intelligent lookout for it, than to run the risk of developing a serious problem through ignorance.

Does everyone who has a family history of diabetes develop it sometime in his life? Luckily, the answer is no. There is a one-out-of-two chance that the children of a diabetic parent will inherit the "diabetic tendency." (The meaning of that term, however, is both vague and complex since by it we are not talking about a single gene, but rather a complex multifactorial set of components, the complex and varying orchestration of which determines not only if, but when, and what type, of diabetes one may develop.)

To begin with, *how common is diabetes?* Well, it is the fifth leading cause of death in the United States. Looked at from the point of view of the living, one out of every 20 people in the U.S. is a diabetic. Look around the next time you're on a crowded subway, or consider the people working in your office. In any group of 20 people, the probability is that there is at least one diabetic, *though he may not even know it.*

What are the chief symptoms of diabetes? In the full-blown picture, we see excessive thirst, excessive urination, and excessive appetite with a paradoxical loss of weight and strength. Often the picture is much less dramatic: unexplained weight loss and having to get up to urinate at night persistently and for no obvious reason related to fluid intake. Often the patient comes to the doctor not because of the primary symptoms of diabetes but because of the symptoms of its complications: blurred or decreased vision, because of its damage to the eyes; fatigue and anemia secondary to the chronic kidney disease associated with diabetes; numbness and losses of sensation due to diabetic nerve involvement; ulcers or gangrene of the feet due to blood vessel disease.

Diabetes is a very complex systemic disease whose most obvious manifestation is a disequilibrium in the body's ability to efficiently use the sugar glucose as a source of energy. As medical research has progressed, it has been learned, however, that there are subtle, but nonetheless important, alterations also present in the body's handling of the other two chief types of food substances: proteins and fats. There have even been some studies that indicate that the primary disturbance may be in the blood vessels, with the various metabolic imbalances being concomitant or secondary to that.

In spite of all these new insights, the practical fact remains that as long as the patient is spilling large quantities of sugar in his urine he is subject to all the complications of diabetes, running from impairment of circulation to gangrene, increased infections, kidney and visual problems, hypertension and coronary artery disease, and early death. The epoch-making and Nobel Prize-winning discovery of the 1920's that the injection of insulin in carefully calculated, specific amounts would help diminish, if not completely control, this spillage of sugar marked the turning point in the history of diabetes. No longer were diabetics required to starve themselves to almost emaciated weights. More balanced diets became possible with the addition of insulin, and best of all, a marked but very significant diminution in the above complications was noted in those who took their injections regularly and were careful in their periodic checks of sugar spillage into the urine.

The time and type of the development of diabetes is very important. There are two chief categories: juvenile diabetes, that usually more serious type, manifestations of which occur sometime before the age of 21 or so (this group makes up about 10% of the almost 10 million Americans who are diabetics), and the second category, the so-called maturity-onset diabetes which usually occurs after the age of 40. While it is true that both types have a hereditary tendency, juvenile diabetes is by far the more serious of the two. It is almost as if the juvenile diabetic makes no insulin at all to metabolize the sugars his body takes in through his diet. As such, the insulin spillage in the urine, the burning up of the normal body tissues in an attempt to supply the body with sufficient energy—the entire picture—is much more serious than is the case with maturity-onset diabetes. Almost invariably, therefore, juvenile diabetics will require daily insulin by injection (it does not work by mouth since it is destroyed by the stomach juices) to keep their disease under control. Maturity-onset diabetics, however, have only a relative deficiency of their insulin production. As a matter of fact, maturity-onset diabetics are usually overweight, and it is almost as if their body has inherited an inability to make up enough insulin to feed and fuel their excess bulk. Often, if they get down to a more ideal weight, their diabetes comes under very significant control. Maturity-onset diabetics do not require, as a rule, the injection of insulin. The very latest approach for their control is to rely completely on diet and weight loss. They should avoid (as is true for just about everyone) the free sugars such as are found in candy, cake, and soft drinks. By utilizing a balanced diet which includes the presence of the starches in reasonable quantities and by avoiding sugars, these diabetics will do quite well if they can control their weight. Between the mid 1950's and the early 1970's, oral antidiabetes medications were widely used to help control the blood sugars of maturity-onset diabetics; however, with the recent demonstrations that these drugs are associated with increased occurrences of the very complications, such as coronaries and strokes, that diabetics were prone to if untreated, the use of such medications as the oral antidiabetes pill has come under fire and is gradually falling into disrepute.

Diabetes, therefore, should no longer be a secret disease. Yes, it may very well be hereditary; yes, it is a chronic disease which cannot be cured; but also, yes, it is a disease for which much can be done to keep it under control and to help assure a good life span for those who are its victims.

DR. VERDESCA'S SLOW WEIGHT LOSS DIET

The question often arises, how does one lose weight if one wishes to do so for medical or just psychological or cosmetic reasons? As all of us who have been or are overweight know, this is far from easy to do; but it can be done—in many ways. Unfortunately, the results, while definitely achievable, are often not permanent. That's one of the reasons for the recurrent popularity of the various fad diets that hit the best seller lists. Though almost all are successful in bringing weight down (even some of the more bizarre and definitely not medically recommended ones), the problem is that within a few months of stopping the diet, the weight begins to creep back up, and in many cases one is back where one started.

One of the basic facts to keep in mind is that every fat person didn't get that way overnight. It took months, if not years, of regular ingestion of more calories than one was burning up in order to accumulate that excess weight. If one keeps that in mind, it helps reconcile one to the concept that the weight loss should be in as physiologic a manner as the weight gain was, that is, slow but steady. Most overweight persons haven't gained 25 pounds in 1 year; therefore, they shouldn't try to lose 25 pounds in 1 year. This is another way of saying that even 2 pounds a month may be too rapid and, therefore, too unnatural, a way of losing weight. One-pound-a-month weight loss is perhaps the lower limit if one wants really to call it a weight loss program. Anyone who has to lose only 4 or 5 pounds doesn't have a really major weight problem in the first place, so much of what follows here is not for him anyhow.

Secondly, and this may be the most important factor to be pointed out, one must almost want to lose weight more than anything else in the world. It requires dedication through thick and thin (pun intended), a willingness to put up with the diet when you are feeling depressed and low and tired, and the courage to turn down a fattening dessert when it has been presented in the most appetizing fashion you have ever seen in your entire life. But, if you really want to lose weight, you will.

O. K.—so you really want to lose weight and you are willing to do it slowly—how do you go about it? "Dr. Verdesca's Slow Weight Loss Diet" would go something like this. Let's say you have decided to lose 1 pound a month (after all that's 12 pounds in 1 year and in 2 years almost 25 pounds, which most people would be very, very happy to settle for). Get yourself an inexpensive weight scale and weigh yourself, undressed, every morning without fail (no jiggling back and forth from one foot to the other is permitted). If you really want to make sure that you are not kidding yourself, get on the scale three separate times each morning with your eyes closed. After you are sure you have stopped all your jiggling, stop moving, open your eyes, take a reading, and settle for that day's weight as the average of those three readings. At the first of each month you have at least 30 days in which to lose the weight. You may by some fortuitous dieting combination do so in 5 days. Fine! Just keep that weight off for the rest of the month, and start on your second pound at the beginning of the next month—not sooner. If, on the other hand, you are coming up on the 25th day of the month and you haven't lost that pound, drastic measures may be in order; but you have got to get that pound off in that month, even if it requires 1 day of almost total starvation (which is indeed very hard to do and not generally recommended because it is not very healthy in the long run anyhow).

Do you avoid carbohydrates? No! Do you avoid proteins? No! Do you avoid fats? No! Just eat a balanced diet every day, but less of it. Of course, for the person who is a sweets-eater, cutting out that form of carbohydrates while still eating his usual complex carbohydrates, such as starches in bread and potatoes, will result in a nice quick weight loss. Many a fattie, however, is not a sweetie: He likes his bread and spaghetti and meat and potatoes, and so then the recommendation is to eat less of everything. True, you have to lose 3,500 calories worth of energy in order to lose a pound but when you buy (in any bookstore) a calorie weight table of foods, you will see how little is required to be omitted from one's diet in order to lose 3,500 calories over a period of an entire month. Warning: Since this is such a slow weight loss, constant vigilance is the watchword. Don't let yourself coast into forgetting that you must continue to watch everything you eat.

This 3,500 calorie a month weight loss really requires a minor but very real adjustment in your basic way of eating. After 10, 20, or 30 months of this adjustment, it becomes a way of life; and you will usually find that you can keep your weight at whatever level you wish afterwards because you have developed new eating habits.

It can be done. It's a pain. It's lonely. It's hungry. But, after a while, it gets to be beautiful when you finally see that you can do it, that the weight is coming off. The satisfaction for this becomes such a positive reinforcing factor that it will help carry you through some of the worse "downs" that you will have throughout the weight loss period.

If you continue to eat a balanced diet throughout your weight loss period, there is really no need for vitamin supplementation. It won't hurt if you take a daily vitamin; and contrary to what everybody in the world knows for sure, a daily vitamin will not increase your appetite and will not make you gain weight.

Fat may be where it's at, but think thin and win.

DIET I

Periodically the question comes up of the validity or potential harm of a new diet that is currently receiving wide publicity. Luckily most new diet fads have two things going for them: In the first place, it's very unusual for a really dangerous diet to obtain wide publicity, and in the second place, so few people really stick to *any* diet for more than a few weeks that even a potentially harmful diet will probably not have been followed long enough to have caused trouble.

Without commenting on any specific diet, it might be of value to review some basic diet information that holds for most people. First it should be emphatically stated that all obesity is not the consequence of gluttony and self-indulgence. Too many overweight people resemble the body-build of someone on either their mother's side or their father's side. This would leave one of two possibilities: Either the person and the relatives he resembles are all gluttons, or else there is a heredity tendency toward a certain body-build almost regardless of what you do about it.

There are, however, lots of "fatties" who got that way because of overeating and to whom dieting is recommended by their doctors. The latter is a point worth emphasizing. Most heavy people who want to lose only 5 or 10 pounds probably don't *need* to do it under a doctor's supervision—although it wouldn't be a bad idea for it to be done under his guidance. But any larger proposed weight loss should not only be done under a doctor's supervision but at his suggestion.

The secret of weight loss is really no secret at all. It goes like this: Each person's body lives on and burns a certain number of calories each day— and this varies from person to person. So long as you take in approximately the same number of calories as you use, you will neither gain nor lose weight. So long as you take in fewer calories than your body burns up each day, you will lose weight. And if you eat more calories than you use up you will gain weight. So, what is the simple secret? This: CALORIES DO COUNT.

Most doctors would recommend a diet that leads to a decrease in one's daily food intake without omitting any one of the three major food classes: carbohydrate, protein, or fat. In other words the diet would remain a balanced diet; there just would be less of it. Such a sensible approach would probably not require any vitamin supplementation—but we still haven't reached the time where people are going to be sensible about dieting. Because of this, I think most dieters should take some form of daily all-purpose vitamins to make sure they don't run into a deficiency state.

The body can store energy in the form of fat, but it has no significant way of storing protein. Yet there are a definite number of essential proteins that the body needs each day. What this all means is that for those who go on unbalanced reducing diets, it is important that regardless of the particular diet they are following, there is a minimal amount of protein that they should take in. The latest U.S. Bureau of Nutrition recommendation is that one should ingest each day 0.9 grams of protein per kilogram of body weight. A kilogram is

2.2 pounds. So, a 154-pound person weighs 70 kilograms and should therefore take in at least 63 grams of protein a day. Now 63 grams of protein is only 252 calories of food—and no one is suggesting that this is all one should eat a day. Rather, regardless of the total calories of one's special diet, one should take in at least that minimal amount of protein per day (not per meal). When one realizes that 1 pound equals 454 grams, then one can see that 60–70 grams of protein is only about 1/6 of a pound of protein in a whole day—and that isn't much. Note that any good form of protein will suffice as this protein source, be it meat, fish, eggs, cheese, milk, chicken, or even vegetable protein.

That represents the absolute minimum of protein that one should have daily. The rest of the ingredients of your diet should be determined by your doctor. What about those people who follow widely publicized diets without seeing their doctors? So long as they take in the minimal amount of required protein and a daily vitamin and so long as the diet is not prolonged for more than 4 to 6 weeks, they probably won't get into any trouble and they probably will lose weight.

DIET II

The question of diet pills comes up regularly. There are two main classes of diet pills: One, more easily discussed, is the so-called water pill. Actually it's an antiwater pill in that it forces the body to lose water and salt through the kidneys. With this fluid loss there is, naturally, some loss of weight, but this is really a trick because no body fat stores are depleted—and that's really where the action is. Also the water pills will only work for a few days because, luckily, there is a limit to how much water and salt the body will allow to be drawn from it artificially. The final clincher is that once one stops the water pills, the body, in the course of the next few days, will reestablish its own salt and water contents and will, therefore, in most cases, now replace all the salt and water that had been drained from it.

The other type of reducing pill belongs to the amphetamine class. These are the "pep pills" one reads about. ("Speed" and "STP" and other popularly-abused drugs also belong to this class so they should be treated with a healthy respect.) Do they work? In most cases, yes.

What's the secret? None. Or, rather, they result in a decrease in food intake and, as always, if you take in fewer calories per day than your body uses, you're bound to lose weight. At one time it was felt that their main effect was on internal metabolism, but this has not been verified. It is true that these pills make one quite restless, restless people more around a lot, and moving around a lot results in energy expenditure with its concomitant calorie loss. But this is only a minor effect. The main effect of the amphetamines is to reduce food intake by acting on the brain. Their actual mechanism of action is not clear, but in some persons, they undoubtedly do lead to weight loss. It's too bad that in our society we need a pill to reduce food intake when we know that that's the only way to lose weight, especially since the pill in question is a drug among whose common side effects are restlessness, dizziness, trembling, talkativeness, tenseness, irritability, and insomnia, with a period of fatigue and depression following the cessation of the drug. Other side effects have included headache, palpitations, irregularities of heart rate, angina, excessive sweating, dry mouth, metallic taste, nausea, vomiting, diarrhea, and abdominal cramps. So not only should the drug be used under a doctor's careful supervision; but second, third, and even fourth thoughts should be given to its use at all.

DIET III

There are a few final topics regarding ways of losing weight that warrant some comment. In the previous article, we discussed the two main types of pills that people take to help them reduce. There is one further medication also used that I have nothing good to say about in connection with weight reduction. The drug I'm referring to is thyroid hormone. It happens to be an excellent, curative medicine for myxedema (deficiency of thyroid hormone) and often is very worthwhile in helping to control and treat goiters. It has, however, no place whatsoever in any sensible program of weight reduction. Any increase in normal metabolism that might result from taking the drug is temporary because the drug will eventually suppress your own natural thyroid hormones so that, in the long run, you're back where you started except now you're taking a medicine every day. It is true that people with overactivity of the thyroid gland produce excess thyroid hormone and often lose weight, but the converse is not true: Underactivity of the gland, or hypothyroidism, does not necessarily lead to weight gain. I personally have never seen a fat person whose basic problem was due to thyroid deficiency. Obesity, in the overwhelming majority of cases, is not due to thyroid abnormalities; and giving thyroid hormone to control it is only to be condemned.

The question of the value of exercise in a program of weight reduction is a difficult one for me to handle because I personally feel that, *as a way of losing weight,* exercise is pretty much a waste of time. The only exercise I would recommend is that old saw about "push-ups": Push yourself up and away from the table whenever you consider second helpings. While it is true that exercise does burn up some calories, here are some of the hard facts: If you walked for 18 minutes, you would use up only 95 calories, which is, for example, the caloric equivalent of one tablespoon of peanut butter. You'd have to swim for 11 solid minutes to burn up the 245 calories of a 3-ounce regular broiled hamburger. Note, this is not the 1/4 pound (4 oz.) hamburger. This is a 3 ounce one. As you can see, you'd have to spend most of your day exercising if you wanted to keep ahead of the calories you'd normally eat. Thus, someone who was eating 2,000 calories a day and who wanted to lose weight by exercising would first have to burn up the 2,000 calories before he could begin to get at his body's stores of fat. To burn up 2,000 calories by walking, one would have to walk for almost 8 hours, or swim for over 3 hours and 40 minutes, or ride a bike for over 4 hours. And after that then one would be just beginning to get down to one's fat stores. You wouldn't have much time to work or do much of anything else except exercise. Obviously, one would be better off eating fewer calories rather than trying to eat one's regular diet and still take off the excess weight by exercise.

One final "Don't" regarding dieting is that it's better not to get fat than to have to go through all the painful struggles to lose it. Therefore, a word to parents: Once you know your child is eating a balanced diet, don't keep insisting he eat, eat, eat because he'll get fat, fat, fat—and the eating habits of a lifetime are often established in childhood. For better or for worse, our society's values are such that obesity is considered undesirable. Therefore, parents would be sparing their children years of loneliness and heartache if they taught them the principles of eating a balanced diet when young and if they cautioned against overeating.

One positive thing that can be said is that quite often the various weight control groups that have been springing up all over the country do work. First of all, the best of these groups recommend sensible diets—which is one of the first considerations in any program of weight control. Second, and probably even more important, is the factor of group interaction. As with A.A. for alcoholics, such groups help to give psychological support to their members and serve continually to point out the problems inherent in good weight-reducing programs. Third is the patient's own resolution. Once he's decided to go through with such a public attempt at weight control, he's probably made the internal decision and commitment to really do something about it and that's really the most important step.

FAT–THIN

Fat is where it's at!! Well, that may be going too far; but while fat may not be "in," it probably shouldn't be "out."

It may very well be that a large part of the opprobrium visited by almost everyone upon the overweight is due to the almost constant medical sermonizing about the evils of being fat. The very words we use are loaded words: "Overindulgence" implies too much of something and, therefore, by definition is a to-be-condemned excess. Although, in the long run overweight may remain an undesirable thing in our society for social and cosmetic reasons, the least the medical profession can do is set right some of the misconceptions for which it may have been responsible.

Up until a very few years ago, doctors believed, and, therefore, preached that being overweight was a significant factor in shortening people's lives and that it led to high blood pressure, heart attacks, strokes, and a variety of other undesirable ills. With the advent of large, carefully controlled, statistical studies in the past decade or so, however, the figures (pun intended) don't bear out all the dire predictions doctors used to make. It is true that if a person has high blood pressure and is significantly overweight, losing weight will help control the blood pressure and thereby improve his over-all "illness-and-death" statistics. If a person has high blood fats and is overweight, certainly weight reduction will help significantly in their control. Similarly, it is most important for a person who is both diabetic and overweight to bring his weight under control as expeditiously as possible in order to achieve better diabetic control and also improve the quite unfavorable "illness-and-death" statistics that way.

All of this notwithstanding, one of the interesting findings of the new statistical surveys is that in the absence of high blood pressure, in the absence of high blood fats, in the absence of diabetes, being overweight *per se* is not associated with any increased prevalence of the diseases we have been warning people about all these years. We are not talking here about gross, massive obesity, but rather we are talking about people who are up to 30% above their ideal weight. The "illness-and-death" statistics for the grossly obese are not good at all.

One other *caveat* might be in order. If one doesn't personally have an elevated cholesterol, or an elevated blood pressure, or diabetes but is indeed overweight *and* has a strong family history of any of the above conditions, then it might be in order for such a person to give serious consideration to weight reduction even though these conditions are not yet present, since the hereditary aspect of these diseases is quite strong. If weight reduction is implemented, the potential expression of these hereditary tendencies might very well be forestalled or held in total abeyance.

It seems as if the medical information about what makes people heavy in the first place is far from all in. Certainly, it is true that calories do count and that when a person is starving, he will lose weight; but it is also true (and many a lean man can testify to this by just looking around at others during meals) that food intake is not the sole factor in determining whether one will become overweight. We all know people who "eat like a horse" but will remain, to the envy of many, "thin as a rail." It can't be just food intake that determines body form.

Perhaps the most important determinant of body form is heredity. Most of us resemble an ancestor or a combination of one or two ancestors, not only in our facial features, but in our body's shape. In other words, just the way the color of our eyes and the color of our hair is inherited, so, in all likelihood, is our ultimate bodily configuration also inherited; and it would be a little foolish, as well as perhaps unfair, to accuse every fat person of secret gorging when his ancestors were built just like him. They can't all have been secret gorgers going on backwards down that family tree.

It may very well be true that a heavy person eats more than most people, but this is the thing that we seem to have missed all along: He probably was eating more than most people all his life and is continuing to eat more than most people even at present. If he was eating more than his body used and this resulted in obesity in the first place, what made his body stop from getting bigger, and bigger, and bigger? Granted that he overate, is overeating, and will continue to overeat, what keeps him from ballooning out completely? Heredity! Once he gets close to the inherited body-build of his ancestors, his body manages to burn up the excess calories probably as efficiently as they are burned up by the skinny guy who "eats all the time and never gains weight."

Some doctors have claimed that the skinny person has a relative metabolic inefficiency in that he is not able to take advantage of all of the calories he ingests, while the fat person has a more efficient metabolism and thus gains weight. We are, nonetheless, left with the interesting paradox that once the fat person attains his inherited body-build, he then seems to develop that same metabolic inefficiency of other large eaters because, obviously, he doesn't keep getting larger, and larger, and larger.

We really don't know the full workings of hereditary factors, but probably part of the way they are expressed is through the intricate and delicate hormonal balance in the body. The old belief that teenagers only eat when they are hungry and only as much as they need and that is why they don't gain weight but stay relatively thin and lithe-looking can be currently exploded by any parent who will tell you that they eat all the time, and in large quantities. The explanation can't only be that teen-agers are "much more active." Some of them are and some of them aren't. Many a paunchy man hides behind "I was thin until I got married, but my wife's cooking is responsible for my gaining weight," when it may very well be that he was eating greater quantities of food when he was a teen-ager than in his now more sedentary middle (pun intended) years.

There may very well be a complex combination of hormonal changes that takes place after one is 20 where now, for example, that family heredity tends to make for the deposition of body fat. Just as male hormones make for muscularity, there are other hormones in the body that are also operative: thyroid hormone, adrenal gland hormone, insulin, and perhaps others that we are not even aware of. One recent study shows that between the ages of 20 and 30, in men and women, the blood plasma level of one of the hormones produced by the adrenal cortex drops off strikingly. So we are not dealing with a hormonal milieu which is very constant throughout one's lifetime. It is probably the decreasing concentrations of certain hormones or at least an alteration in various hormonal ratios as we age that is in large part responsible for the weight gain we see in the middle years.

So, pure and simple obesity in the absence of various other medical conditions may be no more dangerous to one's health than not being overweight. And it is not necessarily true that all overweight people get that way because of gluttony. We all know many a fat person who insists that he doesn't eat that much. After all, have we ever stopped to think that maybe he was telling the truth?

QUICKIE FOODS

The fast-food industry is one of the most rapidly growing industries in the United States today, and it also is coming in for lots of criticism because of the generally assumed lack of adequate nutrition in fast foods. A recent survey indicates, however, that the situation may not be so bad as many people think. The old saying, "better a hot dog in a child's stomach than a steak on his plate," may turn out to be true after all.

This is not to unequivocally defend all roadside-stand type snacks; rather it is to say that all such items are not all bad. If you have a person who, because of some psychological idiosyncrasy, persists in living on candy bars and soda exclusively, he will certainly run into all the consequences of such a nutritionally inadequate diet; but the blame lies with the person and not with the "quickie" foods.

All foods are classified into three main categories: protein, carbohydrate, and fat. For every gram of protein we eat, the body gets four usable calories. That same figure holds for the carbohydrates. When we eat 1 gram of fat, however, the body reaps from it nine calories. In other words, weight-for-weight, fat is more than twice as fattening as proteins and carbohydrates.

The National Research Council has for many years been trying to define a nutritionally adequate diet—all based upon the underlying importance of protein. Protein is the building block of much of the important structures of the human body, and there are actual "essential amino acids" (sub-unit building blocks of proteins) which the body cannot make from ingested fat or carbohydrates or even from other different proteins. What this amounts to is that while it is impossible in any kind of normal diet to avoid all carbohydrates and fats, nonetheless were such a diet achievable, it could very well be nutritionally adequate since a pure protein intake would certainly assure the supply of essential amino acids. On the other hand, a diet which is completely free of protein will always be nutritionally inadequate in the long run.

With these considerations in mind, the National Research Council defined, a number of years ago, the minimum daily adult requirement for protein to be 1 gram per kilogram of adult body weight. One kilogram is 2.2 pounds so an average 150-pound man weighs a little less than 70 kilograms. This would mean that he has to take in at least 70 grams of protein a day for adequate nutritional balance. More recently, however, the National Research Council has determined that 1 gram of protein a day is more than adequate and has lowered the requirement to .9 grams per kilogram a day, and there is recent talk that this may even be lowered to .8 grams per kilogram a day. Sticking with the currently accepted figure of .9, this would mean that the average 150-pound adult needs a minimum of 63 grams of protein a day. At the rate of four calories per gram, this comes to 252 calories of minimal protein intake. The average adult woman ingests about 1,800 calories a day, and most adult men ingest 400 to 700 calories above that, so it's easy to see that in order to have a nutritionally adequate diet, the amount of necessary protein in relation to total daily caloric intake is not very large at all. The rest of the calories can be taken in the form of carbohydrates and fat and will still be nutritionally adequate. A diet of one big steak a day and all the rest in candy bars may not be very good for your teeth and would be most unwise if there is any possibility of diabetes in your background; nonetheless it could result in a nutritionally adequate diet. That is an extreme; but as we examine it closer, it will turn out that the "junk" that our teen-agers and other people eat at quickie food places may, at worse, only be somewhat analogous to that.

It should be emphasized that these 63 grams of protein for the theoretical 150-pound man is not 63 grams at every meal but 63 grams altogether in one day, and that includes all protein sources, be they meat, fish, chicken, eggs, cheese, milk, beans, peas, etc.

Mainly because publicity would have us believe that McDonald's is the largest selling hamburger in the United States, I will use a McDonald's hamburger as an example. One McDonald's hamburger contains, besides a lot of other stuff, 40 grams of protein. Someone who eats two of these a day would be getting, regardless of age, an adequate protein intake. Many of our youngsters about whom we worry so much, weigh considerably less than 150 pounds, and so they need even less than 63 grams of protein a day. Two McDonald's hamburgers would certainly be fine for their total protein intake. Of course, a favorite with many people at quickie food places is a milk shake which is made with milk and ice cream. An 8-ounce glass of milk contains almost 10 grams of protein. A scoop of ice cream only contains about half as much, but the total may be close to 15 grams of protein in a standard milk shake. So, we can see that one hamburger and one milk shake and nothing else during the course of a day would give 55 grams of protein which is almost enough protein for a day, even though it may not be enough for that person in calories.

The only other complaint that one might dredge up against the quickie food stands is the amount of caffeine a person might ingest with the drinking of colas. Noncola drinks usually contain no caffeine, but it is true that cola drinks contain up to 30 milligrams of caffeine. Caffeine is a chemical; it is a stimulant. Used to excess it can indeed make a person "nervous," it can interfere with some people's ability to get to sleep, and it can cause gastric irritation. By "used to excess," I mean more than the equivalent of five or six cups of coffee a day, which is more coffee than most people drink. Since coffee contains an average of 100 milligrams of caffeine a cup, for most people "too much coffee" means more than 500 milligrams a day. Converted into cola drinks, that means more than 15 cola drinks a day. Rare indeed is the human being who drinks that much cola; and if he does, then someone should advise him that he may be taking in too much.

There are, of course, other problems with quickie foods. They are high in fat content; the fat is almost always animal or dairy fat; the foods are often fried in something containing coconut oil, which is very high in saturated fats. A steady diet of these foods, therefore, could certainly contribute to the epidemic of hardening of the arteries, coronaries, and strokes that is afflicting America today; but even that correlation is not completely clear. For people with a high cholesterol or who have a significant family history of coronary heart disease, such steady saturated fat ingestion may indeed be questionable; but for those who do not have these conditions, it is hard to tell them medically that they cannot eat "greasy kid stuff," such as french fries and greasy hamburgers and thick shakes.

One other almost irresistible clincher in favor of quickie foods is: They're cheap.

THYROID CONDITIONS

Even though the once rather faddish diagnosis of "underactive thyroid" has, probably to everyone's good, gradually been diminishing in frequency and in repute, nonetheless thyroid disease, while relatively uncommon, is still a very important aspect of medical practice.

The chief conditions afflicting the thyroid gland are: (1) overactivity, or hyperthyroidism, with or without an attendant goiter; (2) true underactivity which is true hypothyroidism (and not some vague low metabolism as an explanation of the ills of sluggish, slightly depressed, menopausal women or uneasy, middle-aged men); (3) tumors occurring in the thyroid gland—benign and malignant; and (4) a catch-all category, listed as "thyroiditis," including (as the *itis* suffix would indicate) true infections of the thyroid gland, but also comprising some peculiar immune reactions of one's own body against the thyroid gland which, though called "thyroiditis," are not true infections in the first place.

Graves' disease, thyrotoxicosis, and a host of other names are really just among the various titles medicine has given over the years to conditions of thyroid overactivity. The underlying cause has never been completely elucidated. A family tendency is seen in many cases. Certainly true is the fact that the ultimate stimulus for this overactivity of the thyroid probably comes from within the brain itself (even though the thyroid gland is located in the lower front part of the neck) where the "master gland" of the body, the pituitary, is located.

Among the various causes for that pituitary overactivity which causes hyperthyroidism, emotional and/or physical stress have long been accepted as among the most significant. Whatever the ultimate cause, the final result is nervousness, weakness, sensitivity to heat, sweating, restless overactivity, weight loss (usually with increased appetite), trembling of the hands, rapid heart rate, and often an unusual stare and prominence of the eyes.

When such a full-fledged picture as described above occurs, the diagnosis of hyperthyroidism is almost obvious. When, however, only some of the above symptoms are present, there are now available a significant number of rather sophisticated blood tests which can help arrive at the diagnosis. Even radioactivity scans conducted over the thyroid area have proven to be of help. These newer tests are less expensive, easier to perform, and far more accurate than that famous complex breathing test of 30–40 years ago: the basal metabolism test.

Once the diagnosis is established, there are essentially three forms of treatment for overactive thyroids: (1) Chemicals which block or interfere with the massive outpouring into the blood of the excessive thyroid hormone. These are often used first because they do not irrevocably alter the thyroid gland structure itself; and in many cases after 6–12 months of treatment with these medications, they can often be stopped and the patient remains in normal thyroid status. (2) Radioactive iodine in small but very powerful doses is a very popiular form of treatment. The thyroid gland selectively concentrates the chemical, and thus the cell-destroying effect of the radioactivity is confined to the involved gland. Not only is this form of treatment more permanent than the one described above in that it actually results in thyroid gland anatomical destruction, but it can have one rather unpleasant but equally permanent complication: an "overshoot" of the destructive overactivity occurs not infrequently. As a result, the afflicted thyroid gland goes from overactivity into normal activity for a few months and then slips, unfortunately, into true and permanent underactivity. Because physicians are aware that this complication occurs with the use of radioactive iodine, they carefully follow such treated patients to be on the lookout for beginning signs of hypothyroidism. The remedy, taking thyroid hormone replacement pills every day for the rest of one's life, is relatively simple; but, of course, the patient is saddled with a lifetime of taking remedial medications. (3) Thyroid surgery is the other approach to treatment. Once the mainstay of the therapeutic approach to hyperthyroidism, it lost ground for a while when the use of radioactive iodine was in its heyday. With the increasing incidence, however, of irreversible hypothyroidism in a significant number of radioactive iodine-treated cases, surgery has been coming back into its own as, perhaps, the safest, definitive one for the condition. A large part of the thyroid gland can be removed this way, but enough can be left in to supply sufficient thyroid hormone to the body so that subsequent hypothyroidism does not ensue; and because so much of the thyroid gland's hormone-producing tissue has been removed, the likelihood of recurrent hyperthyroidism is generally very remote.

While the above may make it seem as if hyperthyroidism is an "easy disease," it is so only if caught in time and adequately treated. Untreated, it can be very serious, leading to severe debilitation and even heart failure. Some very rare cases of what is called "thyroid storm" have such a massive and overwhelming burst of overactive thyroid activity that the person can literally burn himself up and die of exhaustion if the condition is not treated in time.

Whereas both the picture, the condition, and the treatment of hyperthyroidism are quite clear-cut, hypothyroidism, on the other hand, is a medical morass. Actually, the description of the disease and treatment may be even more clear-cut than in the case of hyperthyroidism. So much confusion, though, has occurred between the combined efforts of patients not being willing to settle for anything less than a "respectable diagnosis" for their tiredness and sluggishness and their doctors' willingness to comply by assigning these problem patients "a slight case of low thyroid" or "a touch of hypothyroidism," that nowadays there is many a person proudly displaying the diagnostic badge of "underactive thyroid" whose thyroid function is, in reality, completely normal.

True hypothyroidism is not a very common disease. As a matter of fact, the most common cause of the condition nowadays is medical; that is, either as a result of a dose of radioactive iodine that inadvertently proved too large for the treatment of hyperthyroidism, or because, again in the treatment of hyperthyroidism, the surgical removal of overactive glandular tissue was too great. In either case hypothyroidism results, and the supplementary intake of hormone is required to restore the patient to normal metabolic health.

True hypothyroidism presents itself as two different diseases depending on the age of the patient. In infants and children the condition can result in cretinism. While cretinism may be caused by a lack of fetal development of the thyroid gland or some kind of complex iodine metabolic disturbance in the fetus, the most common cause of juvenile hypothyroidism is due to prolonged iodine deficiency in the mother and child. This is especially common in certain areas of the world where there is insufficient iodine in the soil and environment, Switzerland being the most famous such area. The introduction of iodized salt has resulted in total prevention of this very serious condition.

For very serious it is indeed. Besides the thick, dry skin, the large protruding tongue, the drooling mouth, the flat nose, the "funny" hands and feet, the pot belly often enclosing an umbilical hernia, the most serious of the manifestations of cretinism is the mental retardation of these afflicted infants. Even in the mildest cases there is minimal retardation, and often it is very severe. If the diagnosis is suspected soon after birth, the administration of thyroid hormone can be of tremendous benefit in restoring these unfortunate children towards a normal status.

Now we come to hypothyroidism in the adult. The full-blown picture is called myxedema and is really an unmistakable medical problem. There is a gradual change in the patient's personality, the face assumes a peculiar pale, waxy puffiness, the tongue actually thickens and enlarges, the speech becomes slow, the voice becomes deep and gravelly, the skin becomes dry and thick, the hands become puffy, the eyelids become swollen, and significant thinning of the hair of the scalp and the eyebrows (especially the outer third of the eyebrows) occurs. Drowsiness, mental apathy, increased sensitivity to cold, and constipation often are found. The heart may enlarge and fluid may accumulate around it. The reflexes become very slow, and a number of blood tests for iodine metabolism become abnormal.

When one sees the rare patient with all those symptoms, the diagnosis is obvious. The problem arises, however, with the so-called early cases. The puffiness of myxedema is a fluid-filled type of puffiness of the tissues and not due to the deposition of fat; therefore, a middle-aged woman who has "become fat for no reason at all" is almost certainly not suffering from hypothyroidism. Nor would a person who's "feeling sluggish" or "has lack of pep" be likely to be suffering from true hypothyroidism. The diagnosis is not a "maybe diagnosis." There have to be very specific abnormal blood tests, or else there is no hypothyroidism. Unfortunately, here the blame must probably be laid largely at the doorstep of the medical profession. A "low normal" blood test does not mean that one is "slightly abnormal." "Low normal" means just that: The person is normal and should not be saddled with the serious diagnosis of hypothyroidism with its concomitant commitment to a lifetime of treatment.

The treatment of hypothyroidism is to replace the body's missing thyroid hormone by any one of a number of compounds, either natural or synthetic. In the case of the person who was normal in the first place but who, nonetheless, had a "low thyroid" diagnosis pinned on him and then was subjected to thyroid pills for the rest of his life, the body luckily knows better than both the doctor and his patient in that it makes the necessary adjustments to keep the patient from suffering from thyroid overactivity caused by the hormone he is taking. Thus, if you never really needed it in the first place because your body was essentially making its normal complement of approximately 3 grains of hormone a day, taking the unneeded 2 grains a day will cause the body to slow down its normal production from 3 to 1, so you will only have a total of 3 grains a day. But, unlucky you in such a case, for now you are stuck with taking a pill for the rest of your life unless your doctor knows enough to wean you off it slowly while the thyroid gland naturally resumes its usual output.

Thyroiditis is an overall term for a number of different thyroid conditions, not all of which (as the *itis* might lead one to believe) are due to infection.

The one that is presumed to be due to an infection of the thyroid gland itself is called subacute thyroiditis. While it has not been proven, the cause is widely accepted as being viral in origin. In support of its infectious nature is the fact that subacute thyroiditis usually follows an upper respiratory infection such as a virus cold or bronchitis. Because the inflamed thyroid gland tends to swell, the patient usually has pain in the neck which sometimes spreads to the jaws, arms, or even the chest. Usually the thyroid gland is firm and very tender. Sometimes the patient has fever, and a number of his blood tests become abnormal. Since the underlying infectious cause is viral rather than bacterial, antibiotics are of no use. However, if the condition is not treated, it can smolder for months, although eventually the patient's thyroid function will return to normal. Aspirin is sometimes used to give the patient relief from the annoying symptoms. If that does not give desired relief, short courses of cortisone compounds have proved satisfactory.

Ignoring some of the other and rarer conditions included under the term *thyroiditis,* one still is left with a fairly common and very mysterious disease: Hashimoto's thyroiditis. Though no one is really sure, it is currently believed that this is one of those peculiar diseases of self-allergy in which the body makes antibodies against its own tissue —in this case, against the thyroid gland. These antibodies then react with, and inflame, the thyroid gland causing the disease. It is not an uncommon disorder: While it is the most common cause of sporadic goiter in children, it is most frequently seen in women of middle age. Further evidence of its being an auto-immune disorder is the fact that it often is found along with one or another auto-immune disorders such as pernicious anemia, lupus, and rheumatoid arthritis. In Hashimoto's thyroiditis, the entire thyroid gland enlarges to a kind of rubbery consistency. First, the patient will have no symptoms, though his thyroid studies will indicate that something peculiar is going on. Eventually, however, the damage progresses to the point where the thyroid gland becomes sub-functional, and the patient will progress from symptoms of low thyroid output to the full-fledged hypothyroidism we have discussed. Since generally there are no spontaneous remissions in Hashimoto's thyroiditis, lifelong treatment with replacement of thyroid hormone is usually necessary.

Thyroid tumors or growths can be classified into two broad categories: thyroid adenomas and thyroid carcinomas. Thyroid adenomas are benign growths (that is, not cancerous) which, however, can cause symptoms because of their size and the pressure that they put on adjacent tissues of the neck. A fairly common characteristic of these benign nodules is that they are metabolically active, that is, they continue to produce thyroid hormone. As a matter of fact, it is not uncommon for them to so compress the rest of the normal thyroid gland that they take over the body's total production of thyroid hormone. Unfortunately, these adenomas do not respond to the exquisite feedback-balance equilibrium that the body maintains between its current level of thyroid hormone and the production of new hormone. These adenomas, though benign from the point of view of cancer, can nonetheless cause symptoms in patients because they are often associated with an unrestricted production of thyroid hormone. It is not at all uncommon, as a matter of fact, to have patients with these benign adenomas slip into full-fledged thyrotoxicosis or hyperthyroidism. Luckily for the patient, the condition responds nicely to the usual treatment for hyperthyroidism, be it surgery or radioactive iodine.

Finally we come to the thyroid carcinomas. These true cancers are of three types. One type, fortunately the rarest, is composed of very wild, highly malignant cells, and affects chiefly the elderly. Called anaplastic carcinoma, it is often rapidly fatal since it spreads widely and is usually resistant to X-ray treatments. The second type is the follicular carcinoma which is also relatively uncommon, but it is one that often spreads widely. Sometimes the patient will come in with evidence of its destructive spread to the lung or bone even before one is aware that there is anything wrong with his thyroid gland. The third and most common form of thyroid cancer is called papillary carcinoma. It tends to occur in two age peaks: between the ages of 10 and 30, and then again in later life. It tends to be a very slow-growing type of cancer and, unlike follicular carcinoma, which spreads widely to distant organs through the blood stream, papillary carcinoma only tends to spread to the nearby lymph nodes where it may remain relatively quiescent for many years. Unfortunately, it is possible for it to "break out" and become more malignant.

The suspicion of thyroid cancer is increased when a patient describes relatively rapid, recent thyroid gland growth which is unaccompanied by tenderness. The thyroid gland is often firm and hard, irregular in outline rather than smooth, and no longer freely movable up and down when the patient swallows. Recently, it has been revealed that patients who received, years ago, X-ray treatment to the neck or head for such conditions as enlarged tonsils or acne have a higher incidence than normal of thyroid cancer in later life. The treatment of thyroid cancer is very complex, involving a combination of surgery and hormone therapy.

UNDERWEIGHT

In the Dark Ages (before 1930) when infectious diseases were still one of the leading killers of Americans, a hidden infection *had* to be ruled out in an examination of those who just couldn't gain weight. Tuberculosis, chronic kidney infections, smoldering infections in the blood—all could drain a person. Even now a regular checkup, including chest X-ray and urinalysis, is needed to help rule out such conditions. Nowadays, in the era of successful treatment of such infections, such an underlying cause for the inability to gain weight is uncommon.

Systemic noninfectious conditions also have to be considered: diabetes, overactive thyroid gland, chronic diarrheas, etc. Again, a regular checkup, including blood tests, can rule these conditions out; and in general they are not a significant factor in the chronic underweight.

At one time, inadequate intake of the proper nutriments was important; however, in our present age of relative affluence, this is rare. A review of one's dietary intake is always an important first step, however, for a balanced diet is of basic importance. If you really want to gain weight, make sure you begin with a balanced diet of protein, carbohydrates, and fats, including meat, fruit, vegetables, and cereals; and then eat excess food over and above that balanced diet.

Most of the above list are rare, and so we're still left with the thin person who, for some unknown reason, can't gain weight. It is very important to know that once conditions such as the above have been ruled out by your doctor, being underweight is itself no cause for concern *unless one had previously been heavier and gradually has lost weight for some unknown reason.* In such instances, a serious condition must be vigorously looked for by your doctor. But the person who was a thin child, a thin adolescent, and now is a thin adult really doesn't have anything to worry about after he's been given a clean bill of health by his doctor.

But there's hope for some of them after all. Marriage sometimes helps. The "thin man" or the "thin girl" will come in, a year or so after being married, no longer thin—but some of them actually getting overweight! What's happened? Regular meals, balanced meals, "good home cooking," keeping more regular hours have turned the trick. But there's another hidden factor: Most people marry before the age of 25, and many people are still growing in their early 20's. So, a fixed food intake that kept you thin and growing may suddenly cause you to gain weight when you've stopped growing.

Hormones must be a factor, but their exact role is unclear. Thus, the thinnest girl will suddenly blossom during pregnancy and, not infrequently, just as suddenly unblossom within a few months of the baby's birth.

Certain male hormones also help keep one thin; thus, men with absolute deficiency of male hormones tend to be very obese. The whole hormonal area is very new and complex, however.

Finally we still have those people who *have* stopped growing, who *do* eat well, get *plenty* of rest, have *completely* clean bills of health from their doctors, who eat like horses, but who still stay thin. For them we really have no answer, but I do have a comment—lucky them! They have inherited the right genes! They can not only eat all they want and still keep slim, but they have better prognoses for long life than the rest of us. They rarely have high blood pressure, they rarely have coronaries, they rarely have strokes—and they generally live longer than the rest of us. So, that particular cloud ("I just *can't* gain weight") has a very silver lining indeed.

VITAMINS

Vitamins are big business. Lots of people take them; most of them don't need them. Most vitamins (but *not* all) have no side effects to speak of so most of us can take them with impunity even when we don't need them.

A vitamin is a chemical that we need for our normal daily metabolism but which is not manufactured to any significant degree by our own bodies and which must, therefore, be supplied by an outside source. Before covering the individual vitamins, one concept which we must keep in mind throughout the discussion is that a healthy person who eats a well-balanced diet receives adequate amounts of vitamins from his food and, therefore, does *not* need any vitamin supplements.

The principal vitamins can be classed in two groups:

1. The fat-soluble vitamins: Vitamins A, D, E, and K.
2. The water-soluble vitamins: Vitamin C and the Vitamin B family which includes thiamine (Vitamin B$_1$), riboflavin (Vitamin

B_2), niacin, the Vitamin B_6 group (which includes pyridoxine), pantothenic acid, folic acid, and Vitamin B_{12} (cyanocobalamin).

Vitamin A

Vitamin A is one of the two vitamins you *can* get too much of—to the point where there is actually a disease called hypervitaminosis A. Vitamin A or its chemical precursor is found in many food sources: the vitamin itself being present only in animal foods such as fish liver oils, liver, egg yolk, butter (plus our modern substitute: Vitamin A-fortified margarine), and cream, while its precursor is present in green leafy or yellow vegetables such as spinach, kale, mustard greens, collard greens, and, of course, carrots.

The chief bodily functions of Vitamin A include the maintenance of the integrity of the photo pigments of the retina of the eye, and thus it is involved in night, day, and color vision; the maintenance of normal skin; the preservation of specific biological membranes deep within the cellular structure of the body; and, perhaps, assisting in the formation of the hormones of the adrenal gland. Some of the principal manifestations of Vitamin A deficiency are night blindness, dryness of the corneal and conjunctival outer layers of the eye; thickening and change of the skin which lines the lungs, the gastrointestinal tract, and the urinary tract; and an increased susceptibility to bacterial infections.

Vitamin A deficiency is, in common with all other vitamin deficiencies in the United States, very rare. Only a person who literally avoided all the foods listed above would become a serious candidate for such a deficiency and, even then, it would require a long period of deprivation before such a deficiency would manifest itself. An interesting question comes up regarding people who go on weight-reducing diets. Often the first things they avoid are such obviously fattening items as butter, ice cream, and fats. Theoretically it's possible if they're not great liver and mustard green lovers for them to run into a mild or sub-clinical deficiency of Vitamin A, not only because they are actually diminishing their intake of Vitamin A-rich foods, but also because they're diminishing their intake of fats in general which, in turn, might decrease their absorption of whatever Vitamin A *was* in their diet, since Vitamin A is fat-soluble and must be in a complex "fatty solution" in order to be absorbed. It is mainly for this reason that I have recommended daily vitamins to those who go on reducing diets: They might help prevent some of the admittedly rare sub-clinical manifestations of Vitamin A deficiency.

Just to remind us of the potency of Vitamin A, a few words about hypervitaminosis A might be in order. Always the result of excess ingestion of the vitamin either in medicinal form as in a vitamin preparation (which is one good reason to keep vitamin preparations away from the hands of curious children) or from the very rare ingestion of food which has *massive* amounts of Vitamin A (such as polar bear or seal liver), hypervitaminosis A will manifest itself in its early form by sparse coarse hair, loss of eyebrow hair, dry rough skin, and cracked lips. Later, severe headache and generalized weakness are added to the picture. Enlargement of the liver and spleen can eventually occur. Finally, especially in children, thickening of the bones and bone pain can occur.

Vitamin D

Vitamin D is the other vitamin you can get too much of, but first let us consider the vitamin in general along with its more common deficiency state. Vitamin D deficiency is the cause of rickets. While the condition is definitely uncommon nowadays, it has been estimated that, in the early 1900's, approximately 90% of the children of northern European cities had rickets.

The principal sources of Vitamin D are fish liver oils, butter, egg yolk, liver, and the ultraviolet irradiation of natural sunlight. (The normal skin contains a Vitamin D precursor that is activated just by getting plenty of sunlight.) The chief functions of Vitamin D are normal metabolism and formation of bone by regulating the intestinal absorption of calcium and phosphorus. Thus, the chief manifestations of deficiency of D are bone problems.

Early rickets in infants can also have generalized symptoms such as unusual restlessness and poor sleep. Such infants do not sit, crawl, or walk early. Then come the obvious bone deformities such as the bowlegs, knock knees, and pigeon breast.

Vitamin D deficiency is not, however, limited to infants. In adults it causes a condition known as osteomalacia which leads to losses of mineralization and of bone density and of strength in the spine, pelvis, and lower extremities. Bowing of the legs along with shortening of the vertebrae can occur.

Hypervitaminosis D can occur in both infants and adults. The first symptoms are mainly nonspecific ones and include loss of appetite, nausea, and vomiting. Later they are followed by excessive urination, excessive thirst, weakness, nervousness, and generalized itching. Kidney function also can be impaired.

Vitamin K

Compared to Vitamin E, Vitamin K may be considered a more important vitamin because without it, the liver is unable to manufacture some very important chemicals required in the blood-clotting process. As a consequence, sometimes very serious bleeding disorders can result from a Vitamin K deficiency.

Vitamin K sources in humans are unique—they come from outside the body, yet one is already inside the body. Vitamin K is found "outside" in such foods as leafy vegetables, pork liver, and vegetable oils. But the chief source, while technically not part of us and therefore "outside" the body—is also inside the body. What I'm talking about are the bacteria in the human intestine.

Bacteria really aren't "part" of us because they can be eradicated by antibiotics, for example, without causing any damage to their human host. But so long as they reside inside us, these bacteria are actively producing Vitamin K from our foods. So, for those eating a balanced diet and not chronically taking antibiotics, there is no need for Vitamin K supplementation.

Vitamin C and the Vitamin B Family

Now we come to that important class of vitamins: the water-soluble vitamins. These include C and the B family. Deficiencies of these are so rare in the United States that many physicians have never seen a case. For example, scurvy is the disease caused by prolonged deficiency of ascorbic acid—which is the technical name for Vitamin C.

Vitamin C is necessary to maintain the integrity of the supporting tissue of blood vessels and muscles as well as being important in bone and tooth growth. Scurvy usually manifests itself by tiny hemorrhages under the fingernails and easily bleeding gums, along with some generalized body symptoms such as tiredness, weakness, irritability, weight loss, and muscular and joint pains.

The dental manifestation can progress to the point where, if untreated, the teeth may actually loosen and even fall out. Luckily, Vitamin C is easy to come by. It's found in citrus fruits, tomatoes, potatoes, cabbage, and green pepper. Even liver has some Vitamin C. But, one final word about Vitamin C: no solid medical evidence exists that massive doses of Vitamin C—so popular as a preventative for the common cold—do any good at all. (Sorry!)

The number of compounds included in the Vitamin B list has varied. At one time, there were as many as 11. Now, the following seven are considered to be the significant group of B vitamins: thiamine (Vitamin B_1), riboflavin (Vitamin B_2), niacin (also called nicotinic acid), the Vitamin B_6 group (which includes pyridoxine), pantothenic acid, folic acid, and cyanocobalamin (Vitamin B_{12}).

Thiamine deficiency causes beriberi, a disease known long before the concept of vitamins was established. Even now, it's a major cause of death in the Far East; and occasionally one still sees it in the United States, especially among alcoholics.

The symptoms of beriberi are wide ranging, running from tiredness, irritability, poor memory, sleep disturbances, and abdominal discomfort to the more serious and specific symptoms of nerve changes in the legs with their resultant numbness of the toes, burning of the feet at night, calf muscle cramps, and pains in the leg. Eventually the reflexes in the legs can be lost, and the muscles can actually shrink.

Beriberi can also affect the brain with, at first, just confusion manifesting itself. But it can go on to coma and death. Finally, beriberi can affect the heart, leading to heart failure. In short, it is a serious disease indeed. And yet, it is so easily preventable with the right diet, since thiamine is found in dried yeast, whole grains, pork, enriched cereal products, nuts, potatoes, beans, peas, and lentils.

Riboflavin is a B vitamin that is necessary for proper growth and tissue function. Among the symptoms of Vitamin B_2 deficiency are pallor, superficial ulcers and scars around the mouth. Red, scaly, greasy changes around the nasal folds, ears, and eyelids have been called shark skin. The cornea of the eye may be affected.

Even a form of anemia can be present in such deficiencies. Riboflavin deficiency is quite rare in the United States because riboflavin is found so widely distributed in nature, for instance, in milk, cheese, liver, meat, eggs, and also in enriched cereal products.

Pellagra is the disease caused by the deficiency of *niacin.* This disease has multiple manifestations: a peculiar scarlet inflammation of the mouth and tongue, burning of the mouth and throat with abdominal discomfort and swelling, and eventually nausea, vomiting, and diarrhea. Besides these gastrointestinal abnormalities, pellagra has skin and brain abnormalities. At first the skin shows a symmetrical blistering, which easily gets infected especially after exposure to sunlight. Eventually the skin can become thickened, deeply pigmented, and scaly.

As for the brain: at first tiredness and irritability, but then confusion, excitability, and delirium can follow. Again, a bad news disease. The preventive: a diet that is rich in liver, meat, fish, beans, peas, etc., and "variety meats" such as hearts, kidneys, liver, sweetbread (pancreas), and brains.

The rare occurrences of *Vitamin B_6* (pyridoxine) deficiency are manifested by a greasy kind of skin change, inflammation around the lips and tongue, involvement of the nerves of the extremities, and a lowering of one of the protective elements of the white blood cell count.

While most doctors feel that *pantothenic acid* is a real vitamin in the sense that we really need it from an outside source, no clear-cut deficiency picture has been associated with its lack. Some esoteric benefits noted after its administration have included alleviation of the burning or electric-foot syndrome noted in prisoners in World War II and an improvement in the ability of well-nourished subjects to withstand the stress of immersion in cold water. The vitamin is found in dried yeast, eggs, "variety meats," or legumes.

Folic acid and *Vitamin B_{12}* deficiency are chiefly associated with a special form of anemia. Added to the basic anemia they both have in common, Vitamin B_{12} deficiency (pernicious anemia) is associated with severe disturbances in the nervous system.

Folic acid is found in fresh green leafy vegetables, fruit, "variety meats," liver, and dried yeast while Vitamin B_{12} is found in liver, meats (especially beef and pork), eggs, milk, and milk products.

Let me close by saying that Vitamin B_{12} is not good for anything except preventing pernicious anemia.

Vitamin E

A headline in a very reputable newspaper read: "Vitamin E New Fad—Only Lack is Popularizer of Pauling's Eminence." Luckily, a Linus Pauling (the most recent popularizer of Vitamin C) has *not* yet come along. Many articles have appeared heralding the benefits of Vitamin E: Most have appeared in the popular press of newspapers and magazines; some, unfortunately, have even appeared in some medical journals. I state "unfortunately" because in no instance have such articles been based on the sound science of careful statistics and controlled clinical trials; they really have been little more than enthusiastic personal endorsements.

Generally speaking, in medicine one will find that an active drug or medication usually has a relatively narrow spectrum of specific clinical application. Anything that "works" for a wide-ranging variety of totally unconnected diseases is either one of the most unusually potent medicines of all time (of which there are very, very few examples) or else probably doesn't work at all—and owes its popularity to Western man's almost incurable attraction to pills and medical fads.

Thus, large doses of Vitamin E have been claimed to be efficacious in preventing habitual abortions, curing sterility, in coronary, cerebral, and peripheral vascular disease, in various muscular dystrophies, and also for nocturnal leg cramps. It's also supposed to improve the control of diabetes, retard the aging process, cure impotence, and speed the healing of wounds and burns, besides being of help in high blood pressure, peptic ulcers, and kidney disease. That list alone should make one suspicious of the whole Vitamin E picture. To add to the confusion, the Vitamin E boosters disagree among themselves. Thus, recently an entire book was published extolling the marvelous cardiovascular effects of Vitamin E. The author then goes on to categorically deny one of the most popular of all the "cures" that are attributed to Vitamin E: He specifically and carefully disclaims any effect of Vitamin E in enhancing sexual potency!

Vitamin E is a fat-soluble vitamin that was discovered in 1922, when it was found to be a necessary item in the diet of female rats if they were to reproduce normally. (However, the jump from mice to man doesn't necessarily follow.) It was first isolated in 1936 from that other reputed "wonder of nature"—wheat-germ oil. Since that time Vitamin E has become recognized as an essential factor in the diet of many mammals, various species of birds, and at least one species of fish. Vitamin E lack, in *these species,* does produce signs and symptoms that are relieved or cured by reexposure to the vitamin.

This does *not* hold true for man. In fact, there is no well-defined Vitamin E deficiency state in the human adult. The absence of such a deficiency state makes it very difficult to come up with any meaningful guidelines for a daily dosage requirement for the vitamin. In the case of the other vitamins that humans need, the recommended dietary allowances are based on the actual requirements for the vitamins as shown by their ability to prevent or cure a specific deficiency state. In the case of Vitamin E, however, since there wasn't really any definable deficiency state, what was done was simply to calculate the range of intake of Vitamin E that most people have each day and then to declare *that* figure was the recommended daily allowance. "Curiouser and curiouser."

It's almost impossible to avoid Vitamin E in any sort of reasonably balanced diet. Thus, among the sources of naturally-occurring Vitamin E are vegetable oils such as wheat-germ oil, soybean, cottonseed, and corn oil. Vitamin E is also found in fruits and vegetables, in cereals and whole-grain products, and even in egg yolks. (There are only very small amounts of it in meat, however.)

The question that might next arise is: "Well, if it doesn't seem to be any good for those conditions, is Vitamin E good for anything at all?" The answer to that is a soft "yes".

The red blood cells of animals and humans, when test-tube tested for fragility *outside* the human body, were shown to have a greater fragility when drawn from those deficient in Vitamin E than when drawn from those who were not so deficient. But, except for premature infants, such an increase in red blood cell fragility has not been demonstrated to occur in the human body itself. In the test tube, yes; in the body, no. Therefore most specialists do not believe that a Vitamin E deficiency has any adverse blood effects in adults. One study has shown that *very small* premature infants who were fed a commercial formula of skimmed cow's milk and vegetable oils did have this increased red blood cell fragility.

A very rare disease indeed is one called porphyria cutanea tarda. It has recently been shown that Vitamin E may be helpful in its treatment. An even rarer disease is acanthocytosis, which is an inborn error of metabolism. Once again, in it, Vitamin E has proved to be helpful.

Studies to show its efficacy in preventing or controlling other blood disorders, repeated abortions, sterility or any neuromuscular or cardiovascular disease in man have been all negative. The American Heart Association recently concluded, "Massive doses of Vitamin E are neither toxic, nor do they exert any recognizable preventive or therapeutic effects on cardiovascular disorders."

ACUPUNCTURE AND THE POWER OF POSITIVE THINKING

Acupuncture, witchcraft, Vitamin B_{12}, hypnosis, faith healing, doctors, voodoo, and the power of positive thinking—what could they possibly have in common? From the medical point of view, they have the most important thing possible going for them: they work.

I recently unleashed a storm of controversy—or better, a tempest in a teapot—when at some talks I gave, I said that Vitamin B_{12} was good only for pernicious anemia. Then the testimonials started to pour in from people who got Vitamin B_{12} for nerves, to keep their skins from aging, for "that rundown feeling," to help them gain weight, to keep up their resistance while they lost weight, to recuperate from prolonged illnesses, for arthritis, for bursitis, and on, and on.

I wasn't saying that Vitamin B_{12} didn't work in the sense that it failed to make patients feel better. What I was saying—and am here repeating—is that unless they were suffering from a specific deficiency of the vitamin, there was no medical indication for its use, regardless of what condition they were being treated for.

There are only a few conditions for which B_{12} is indicated, the chief and most common of which is pernicious anemia. Yet, pernicious anemia is a relatively rare disease, and the other conditions requiring the vitamin are even more uncommon.

What about regular anemia? Underweight conditions? Arthritis? Bursitis? My answer is, "What about them?" The fact that people swear they were helped by Vitamin B_{12} is indisputable. Well, if the B_{12} didn't help them, what did? The power of positive thinking. They went to the doctor fully expecting help; the doctor examined them and gave them something, and they felt better. This, plus their "mind-set" that something would be done for them, is what made them feel better.

One of the great mysteries of medicine—and yet an undeniable fact —is that surgical procedures can be performed under hypnosis. We don't know just how the mind can control the pain of surgery, or, more mysteriously, not feel the pain in the first place, but it happens. Hypnosis works! So, does acupuncture work? Why shouldn't it? If you can perform an operation just by hypnotizing a person, without sticking anything into him, then I see no reason why poking a few needles into him shouldn't also work. You set the mind (and who knows what that means in medical or chemical terms) and the rest follows.

Recent studies have also shown the real power of voodoo. People do die from it. Autopsies have been performed on such persons without finding any medical cause of death. If you come from a culture where belief in the effectiveness of voodoo is prevalent, and if you really believe in it yourself, then somehow the mind-set takes over and it works. We don't know how, but again we see the great power of the mind over the body.

Faith healing undoubtedly works. Persons whose religious beliefs are such that they resort to faith healers rather than orthodox physicians are not known as "those people who die young." They live as long as the rest of us—without doctors, without medicines, but with the capability we all have: mind-sets toward health.

Witchcraft does not cure tuberculosis. Streptomycin and INH do. Acupuncture does not cure heart failures. Digitalis does. Faith healing does not remove a lung cancer. Surgery does. People have accused me of not believing in medicines. Of course I believe in medicines. What would we do about infectious diseases today if it were not for antibiotics? What would we be able to offer persons with pernicious anemia if it weren't for Vitamin B_{12}?

Perhaps we can put the whole thing together, thus: Medicine has been a respected profession for centuries, long before we had antibiotics or insulin or digitalis or modern surgical techniques—or Vitamin B_{12}. It was respected when it was in the "eye of newt and toe of frog" phase, when doctors listened to your story, examined you, and then applied leeches. Why was it respected? Because it worked, it showed results, most people got better.

What happened to those with pneumonia or heart failure or diabetes?

Many of them died because the right medicines just weren't available. (As a matter of fact, the reason the 20th century has witnessed the dramatic inroads made against the killing diseases is that, at last, the right medicines have become available.) But the overwhelming majority of persons who go to a doctor do not have diseases for which penicillin or insulin or digitalis or Vitamin B_{12} are specifically indicated. These people did well with traditional European medicine, and so it was respected. In other parts of the world, they did well with acupuncture, and so that was respected. And they did well with their witch doctors, and so they were respected.

Two of the most important things in achieving a return to health are the proper mind-set (the power of positive thinking) and the person of the physician. If you believe in doctors, then doctors work. Let no one underestimate the mysterious power of the person to whom you can go when you are feeling bad, when you ache, when you're afraid. That he listens in confidence; that for a brief while, you are the center of his attention; that he cares; that he does something for you: These are of incalculable value and cannot be replaced by a thousand lab tests or a million medicines.

12

Neuro-Psychiatric

DIZZINESS

Dizziness is a common complaint whose causes run from the unknown, through the not-too-serious, to the very-serious-indeed.
Luckily the majority of cases fall into the first two categories, especially the "not-too-serious" category. While "unknown cause" is a
relatively unsatisfactory conclusion, it's better to have dizziness of
"unknown origin" that recurs sporadically for 20 years than to have
dizziness of short duration due to a very serious cause.

First, what is dizziness? It is *not* faintness. It is *not* light-headedness. It is *not* slight swaying. These are merely *physiological* symptoms that can be caused by such things as getting up out of bed too
quickly, or the sudden resumption of the upright position after prolonged squatting, or the lightheadedness and actual fainting that may
occur from too-prolonged motionless standing (as in the case of
soldiers standing at attention on parade grounds). All of the above
are exaggerations of normal body reflexes which are operative in all
of us at some time or other.

True dizziness is a *pathological* symptom. It means something is
wrong with a person's equilibratory apparatus. The truly dizzy person suffers from vertigo which is a feeling of whirling (usually the external world seems to be whirling around the person), or is a feeling
of up-and-down motion or side-to-side motion. In other words, in
contrast to light-headedness or faintness in which some peculiar feel-

ing seems to be present in one's head, in true dizziness something seems to be wrong with the steadiness of the environment.

Every person who first experiences the onset of true dizzy spells should be given the benefit of a thorough history and complete physical examination—which is then followed by an ear, nose, and throat evaluation, a hearing evaluation, and sometimes an X-ray evaluation. The reason the evaluation finally focuses on the ear region is that true dizziness often turns out to be due to some affliction of the vestibules which are bilateral organs of balance located deep in the inner ear. They are not the sole organs of balance, however, for they have nerves leading to specific sections of the brain; and the problem could also lie in those nerves or the brain itself. Even the eyes and their nerves and brain connections are involved in maintaining one's balance.

Among the brain afflictions that can be responsible for true dizziness are some strokes and certain internal brain tumors. Multiple sclerosis is a not uncommon cause, while the brain damage due to syphilis as a cause has become extremely rare, thanks to the advent of antibiotics. A unique form of brain tumor called an acoustic neurinoma, located not so much *in* the brain as at the base *of* the brain, is *usually* associated with true vertigo; and its presence must always be considered a possibility.

Other non-ear causes of dizziness would include the partial or complete closure of a blood vessel at the base of the brain, or some vascular abnormality of the ear or brain.

All of these are potentially very serious conditions and, luckily, are not the *common* causes of dizziness.

More common than the above are conditions associated with the ear, one of the most common of which is Meniere's disease or syndrome. I've not listed this first because it is not true that *every* case of dizziness is due to Meniere's disease. Not every patient with Meniere's disease will have all three of the following symptoms at first, but all of them should eventually experience: (1) attacks of whirling vertigo, (2) ringing in the ear (called tinnitus), and (3) some degree of hearing loss. These persons have isolated attacks of severe whirling vertigo with no dizziness or instability between attacks. The attacks usually begin suddenly but not so suddenly that the patient falls. Typically, the attack gets worse and worse during the first hour, persists unchanged for several hours, and then subsides. Meniere's vertigo lasts for hours, not days or weeks. Some persons may experience nausea and vomiting with their attacks of dizziness. If untreated, Meniere's dizziness episodes tend to become more frequent, going from months apart to sometimes as often as once a week or even every few days.

Some of the other "ear" causes of vertigo include such things as entrapped wax or foreign bodies in the external ear canal—especially if it's packed tight against the eardrum itself. Generally this produces only mild dizziness. Negative pressure in the middle ear which is due to blockage (usually due to a cold) of the Eustachian tube also can cause dizziness.

Acute and chronic middle ear infections can cause mild vertigo, but quite severe vertigo can result if the infection extends into the mastoids.

Even injuries to the ear can cause vertigo. Thus a sharp blow with the open hand may rupture the eardrum and dislocate the three middle ear bones.

HEADACHE

Is there anyone in the world who can honestly say he has never had a headache? Generally, tooth pain, facial pain, even throat and high neck pain, all are probably associated with problems arising in the head somewhere, and yet common, as well as medical, custom would tend to exclude all of these types of pain from the generic term *headache*. Granting the exclusion of all of these, nonetheless, is there anyone in the world who has never had a headache?

Headache means pain in the cranial vault somewhere. There are many ways to approach it. One way is to describe the nature of the discomfort: a steady pain versus a throbbing, beating, pulsatile pain. The latter type of headache (and the classic example of this is migraine) is caused by a problem in the blood vessels inside the head. In migraine, the blood vessels, having been in spasm for too long a time, suddenly are totally paralyzed, so to speak; and the blood comes pounding through in a pulsation synchronized with the heartbeat. Another much rarer type blood-vessel problem causing throbbing headaches would be an aneurysm or a stretching out of the walls of the involved blood vessels. Still another cause is fever: It probably causes dilation of the blood vessels throughout the body, including the head; and whether the blood vessel is dilated because it is almost paralyzed as in migraine, or whether it is dilated because of the toxic effects of the high fever, nonetheless the effect on the structures inside the head is the same: a pain due, so to speak, to the throbbing rush of blood as it is pumped out of the heart. As a matter of fact, some causes of throbbing headache have nothing to do with the unusual dilation of the blood vessels but have to do with the unusual pressure with which the blood is being pumped out of the heart. These would be the headaches that one usually finds in patients whose high blood pressure is poorly controlled.

Though migraine is common, nonetheless throbbing headaches do not make up the majority of headaches. Most people suffer from a specifically localized steady type of pain when they are complaining about headaches. Let's work from the outside in. Pain over the forehead or above the eyes, especially towards the end of the day, and very especially if it occurs in a youngish person such as a teen-ager, is often a manifestation of eye strain. Either the person needs glasses, which is usually the case in the youngsters, or the person's present prescription is inadequate, usually for reading, and this usually occurs in older people. It is generally noted that if a nearsighted person spends a lot of time trying to look off into the distance through glasses that are not strong enough, he generally does *not* develop headaches. On the other hand, if a farsighted person tries to concentrate on reading through glasses which are no longer adequate enough to make the print clear, he will amost invariably develop headaches.

Another cause of *headache* is certain internal ear problems. Infections in the ear itself or in the nearby mastoids can cause one-sided headaches which are often peculiarly stabbing and throbbing in character. Of course, the usual associated fever and/or ear pain is a clue to this type of problem.

Often blamed, but probably not so often guilty, for headaches is sinus infection. Sinus infections can cause headaches under the cheekbones (and, therefore, by our above definition, not truly headaches), but they can also cause pain in the forehead or behind the eyes, at the top of the head, and in some rare cases even at the back of the head. Generally these sinus headaches are worse in the morning, better in the afternoon, often on one side of the face, and usually associated with obvious nasal and postnasal discharge.

A vague category of headaches are the so-called posttraumatic headaches. A person has an injury in which his head gets banged, and usually one would expect the person to have discomfort for a couple of days and indeed he will; but some people continue to have headaches long after the effects of the acute injury will have completely vanished. The fact that such headaches are often made worse by emotional disturbance and are often associated with irritability, insomnia, and inability to concentrate generally leads the treating physician to suspect that there may be a strong emotional factor involved in the underlying cause. Since, however, a small but very significant percentage of headaches can be due to very serious problems, one has to rule out these serious problems in almost every persistant headache, even if the physician suspects that it may be of an emotional origin. Skull X-rays, electroencephalograms (EEG's), and spinal taps are sometimes necessary. Even psychological studies may have to be consulted to help find the cause.

One nonpsychological cause of continued posttraumatic headaches is the presence of what is called a subdural hematoma. What happens in such cases is that the injury is associated with the breakage of a blood vessel in the skull. This continues to leak until the blood clots, leaving behind a clot sometimes the size of a nickel and sometimes the size of a lemon. Naturally, the latter will cause chronic pressure on the brain structures themselves and lead to headaches, probably due to the fact that there is an increase in the total pressure inside the head itself.

When a headache is secondary to an increase in the total pressure of the head contents, generally a serious condition is to be suspected. Since the skull is a very rigid structure, a new growth, leaking blood which then clots, or any other space-occupying lesion cannot cause any expansion of the skull but instead presses inward on the nearby brain structures and at the same time causes a significant increase in the internal brain pressure which, of course, causes a headache. Such headaches are very treacherous because they can mimic almost every other type of headache. Thus, they can be mild, they can be severe; they can be localized or generalized; some may be sudden, some are only intermittent. Generally, however, they are not of the throbbing, vascular, nature such as we described earlier in this article.

Some of the causes of these increased intracranial pressure headaches include things like brain tumors. Tumors originating in the brain are relatively rare, but tumors spreading to the brain from cancers elsewhere in the body are not at all rare and generally herald the fact that the cancer has slipped away from control.

Just as one can have infections in the lungs, in the sinuses, on the skin, so it is possible to have an infection in the brain itself. Such brain abscesses cause headache by the increased intracranial pressure method just outlined. Usually, however, one can find a focus of infection nearby, such as in a sinus or ear infection. Sometimes, though, the source of infection can be remote, such as from a pneumonia or even an infection of one of the heart valves.

A very important class of increased intracranial pressure headaches that is not due to an expanding, space-occupying lesion is the type of headache caused by irritation of the thin linings that cover the brain and spinal cord. The most common cause of these inflammations are those infections which we term *meningitis* (from *meninges,* which is the name for those thin sheaths covering the brain). Acute meningitis headaches are severe and generalized. The headache is sudden and often spreading down the neck so that the person will usually have difficulty in flexing his head. Usually there are obvious signs: fever, vomiting, etc., which lead the physician to the correct diagnosis; but acute meningitis is always a very serious condition which needs the prompt and frequently prolonged application of antibiotics.

There is such a thing as a chronic form of meningitis. This is usually the result of diseases, such as fungus infections, tuberculosis, and syphilis. Here the headache is severe to dull; and the symptoms of acute meningitis are, of course, much less prominent.

Another category of headaches is due not to changes going on inside the skull but to changes of the skull itself. Thus, Paget's disease is an affliction of the bones of the skull. They change, get thicker, become more concentrated, and enlarge, all of which lead to often severe headaches of a burning nature. They may be either intermittent or sudden, localized or generalized. Of course, the patient will usually notice that he has experienced a change in the size of his skull. In this same category of skull problems themselves, some cases of cancer spread not to the brain but to the bones of the skull and, of course, with the destruction of the bones, there will be pain.

Perhaps one of the worst forms of headache is something called trigeminal neuralgia. This lightninglike, stabbing, gasping type of pain which can sometimes even follow a cool breeze on one's face is due to a basic irritation of the nerve coming out of the brain itself. It is still not yet generally known whether this is due to an infection of the nerve from some type of virus, a displacement of the nerve by an abnormal blood vessel, or what; but it can be one of the most crippling forms of headache known to man.

Yet another category of headaches is that which occurs towards the end of the day or after long periods of driving. These headaches are localized along the back of the neck and radiate up to the back of the skull. These are the typical "tension headaches." What is meant by that is that the muscles on the outside of the skull are chronically tense for a number of hours and, as a result, begin to ache. A good night's rest almost invariably relieves tension headaches.

In spite of this long list, nonetheless there are many doctors who believe that most peoples' headaches don't lie in any of the above categories. Rather they would classify them in that vast sea of the unknown: "psychogenic headaches." What they mean is that there is no cause they can find. The patient usually manifests obvious psychological tension in other areas of life, work, etc.; and the headache seems to represent one more manifestation of the underlying tension of the personality rather than a basic affliction of the person. Aspirin by the ton, tranquilizers by the billion, psychiatrists in the millions of dollars, TM, yoga, acupuncture, prayer, and fasting—everything has been tried. Everthing works; nothing works; what works for one person is not good for another and vice versa.

Trying to find the underlying cause of a person's headache is often, for the treating physician, a real headache.

HEAT STROKE AND OTHER HEAT DISORDERS

Probably the most common of these ill effects is the so-called heat faint which may range from simple lightheadedness, all the way through severe fatigue, to actual loss of consciousness. What usually happens is that hot weather causes the blood vessels to dilate; as a result, blood pools in them and blood pressure falls, sweating occurs, the pulse goes up, and, especially if the person has been exercising, the body temperature may actually rise a few degrees. All symptoms subside in a few minutes to an hour if the patient is removed from the hot surroundings and allowed to lie down and rest.

Next in order of severity is heat exhaustion. This takes a few days of unremitting heat exposure to develop. Basically it is due to loss of body salt and water. Early symptoms include headache, fatigue, confusion, and drowsiness. Lack of appetite may be noted; there may be visual disturbances. On occasion, even vomiting may occur and if it persists, may actually lead to collapse of the circulation., Rarely does the picture progress this far, since the patient is usually incapacitated early in the course of the condition and thus obtains treatment before any serious or even fatal consequences can occur. Treatment includes removal of the patient to cool surroundings, rest in bed, and replacement of salt and water.

Heat stroke is probably the most dangerous of the heat disorders. Basically the body's ability to radiate or lose heat is lost. As a result, sweating ceases, the body temperature goes to 105 or 106 and convulsions or coma may follow. Besides the cessation of sweating, other preliminary symptoms can include headache, numbness and tingling, dizziness, restlessness, and even mental confusion. Usually both the pulse and blood pressure are elevated. The hallmarks of the condition, however, are lack of sweating, high fever, and coma. Treatment must be given to avoid brain damage due to the high fever. Cold water or ice baths or wrapping wet sheets around the person, rest, and sedation are essential. If the person cools off too rapidly, vigorous massage of the arms and legs may be necessary to avoid stagnation of blood in the extremities. Temporarily the temperature should not be allowed to fall below 102–103.

Heat strokes, though relatively rare, may be fatal. Even in treated cases, 20–30% may die. Usually the higher the fever, and the longer it has been present, the worse it is for the patient. Ideally the temperature should be brought below 104 within the first hour, and the patient must be watched for at least 24 hours to make sure a secondary rise in temperature does not occur. Sometimes a whole week is needed for the body temperature to stabilize and for sweating to return to normal. If treatment is delayed for more than 4 hours, even though the patient survives, there may be residual lung, brain, heart, liver, or kidney damage.

To prevent heat strokes, one should keep in mind the type of environments in which this illness has occurred or is likely to occur, keep activity down to within safe limits of exposure within this environment, and if one knows in advance one is going into such an environment, allow the body plenty of time to acclimatize itself. Acclimatization needs at least 5 days to occur and is manifested by (even though in a hot environment) lowering of the pulse and rate of respiration, lowering of the body temperature, and an *increased* volume of dilute sweat. Such changes of adaptation are usually complete within 2 weeks and can be maintained by continued periodic exposure.

Finally there is the problem of heat cramps. This relatively mild condition is due to an imbalance in the minerals of the body, usually caused by drinking large quantities of water in a hot environment during sweat-producing work. In essence, this dilutes the body fluids; heat cramps are, therefore, really a form of water intoxication. There is twitching and even spasm of the muscles of the arms and legs and abdominal wall. Usually it occurs late in a workday and is corrected by replacement of salt, in the form of salt tablets. To prevent the condition, extra use of salt is advised for those having to work hard in high temperatures rather than limiting the intake of water since drinking less may prevent cramps but might result in some of the more serious conditions mentioned above.

LSD AND MARIJUANA

LSD is legally an experimental drug, and possession and use of it by unauthorized personnel is illegal. That's what the law says, and if people did what the law says, there'd be no need to write this article. Unfortunately, the illegal use of LSD is not uncommon—especially among the younger half of our population.

While the use of heroin is generally conceded to be a sign of a "hard core" drug addict, the use of LSD or marijuana is often labelled as "experimental"—and somehow this frightens people less. Unfortunately the medical side effects of LSD can be even worse than those of heroin, even though LSD does not seem to be truly addicting.

Except for some recent experimental trials in special glaucoma patients or in special asthmatic patients, marijuana or "pot" is a drug with little proven medicinal use but with some serious medical side effects; it tends to produce hallucinations as well as marked alterations in brain function. Its chief effect is, in fact, on the central nervous system where a combination of excitement (feeling high) and depression (feeling down) is produced. Ordinary consciousness is affected with resultant disconnected, uncontrollable, and rapid ideas. Distance, sounds, and perceptions of time and space can be markedly distorted. Rather than fostering physical intimacy, the reverse is usually true.

A dangerous effect of marijuana is the slowing of reflexes which, combined with the distortion of space and time it produces, is frequently a cause of automobile accidents.

LSD, like marijuana, is not truly addicting; but there the resemblance virtually ceases. LSD is a much more dangerous drug. Perhaps the most frightening of the complications of its use is psychosis, or, in lay terms, "insanity." This is not just a temporary insanity lasting for hours or even a few days. It has, in a number of cases, gone on for months and even years and has resulted in permanent institutionalization. Luckily this is a relatively rare complication, occurring mainly in those whose personalities already had a predisposition toward instability.

LSD differs from most other drugs because its effects occur at varying periods after the injection of the drug, long after the drug has left the blood stream.

While psychosis is a rare complication, impairment of judgment and a reduction in responsibility are common, so much so that one medical source suggests that it is inadvisable for an individual who takes even one dose of LSD to make a major decision about himself for at least 3 months.

Under LSD one tends to ignore facts previously held as valid and, instead, is prone to construct new beliefs no matter how irrational. One may feel he has new powers or has new invulnerability (from this feeling has stemmed the jumping out of windows one reads about). In many respects, fantasy is substituted for reality, with subsequent diminution in real personality output be it work or artistic creations or just normal everyday personality functions such as effectively communicating with others.

A very disconcerting complication of LSD has been reported: It has an effect on the genes that make up each human cell and that we pass on as our chemical heredity.

In short, medical opinion is that while neither marijuana nor LSD is addicting, they are nonetheless very dangerous drugs—to be avoided by everyone.

MIGRAINE

"I'm having one of my migraine headaches." How often one hears such a statement, and how often medical evaluation indicates that the patient is not suffering from migraine after all.

Migraine headaches are recurrent attacks of throbbing headaches, with or without associated visual and gastrointestinal disturbances. They usually begin between the ages of 10 and 30 and very often diminish in frequency after age 50. The condition is much more common in women than in men; and in over 50% of the patients, a family history of the condition can be uncovered.

The condition derives its name from the Latin *hemi-cranium* which was contracted over the centuries to *migrania* and eventually *migraine*. As the name implies, the headache is usually limited to one side of the head, and quite often, it's the same side each time.

While the majority of other types of headaches can occur at any time, migraine headaches usually begin in the early morning hours so that the patient frequently awakens with the headache. Not infrequently the headaches will occur on a Saturday morning or on the first day of vacation or the first "relaxed" day after a prolonged period of tension. Migraine headaches are further distinguished by the fact that they often have a "warning signal" that precedes the actual headache. This can be visual such as bright spots in one half of the field of vision, or zig-zag colored flashes, or rarely even transient blind spots. Other people may have a preceding loss of appetite; others have a sense of confusion or irritability or restlessness.

Although such preliminary symptoms do not occur in all migraine sufferers, they help to make the diagnosis when they *do* occur. They are also of some value to the patient since, if he takes his medication during the warning period, he may prevent the attack itself from occurring.

Characteristically the migraine headache is a throbbing, pounding headache rather than a constant one. As the warning signal (when present) subsides, the one-sided dull, boring, throbbing headache begins, gradually increasing in intensity until the whole of the same side of the head is affected. This much is fairly common to both sexes. The rest of the symptoms occur more often in women than men.

Once the headache has settled in, the patient may feel so prostrate, so nauseated that he can get relief only in a quiet, darkened room. Sometimes vomiting occurs and, peculiarly, it sometimes heralds the end of the headache. Others find that if they can fall into a deep sleep, they'll awaken with the headache gone.

An untreated attack of mirgaine may last from hours to days, and attacks can occur from everyday to once every few years.

The cause of migraine is a mystery. There certainly is a strong hereditary factor in most sufferers, but many people with migraine also have a certain type personality that may contribute to the causation. Thus, in general, migrainous persons are hard-driving, careful, meticulous, neat, expecting much of themselves and very often delivering top-quality work. Yet there are people with such characteristics who don't have migraine, and not all migrainous people are like that.

Luckily there is medicine for migraine: A combination of caffeine and the ergot alkaloids—especially if taken early in the attack—can get rid of it. There's no cure although there is a relatively new medicine which, if taken regularly, can diminish the frequency of the episodes. Unfortunately, some persons have developed some serious side effects to the latter medicine.

In brief, migraine is not just any old headache. It's a very special type of headache, often occurring in a very special type of person, and if caught in time, having a very specific cure.

MULTIPLE SCLEROSIS

Multiple sclerosis remains one of the great mysteries of medicine. We don't know its cause; we don't know why it has such an unusual course; and we don't know its treatment. Let's review now some of the things we *do* know about it.

It is one of the most common of the chronic neurologic diseases; yet, in spite of that and the thousands of doctor-years that have been spent in research, its cause still remains unknown. Attempts to prove that it is due to an infectious organism such as a bacterium or a virus have proved fruitless. Nor have toxic factors such as metallic poisons proved to be a factor. No factor of internal metabolism or blood vessel disorder or injury has yet been shown to be a reliable precursor of the disease.

We do, however, know some seemingly unusual facts about its occurrence. Multiple sclerosis is rare in warm climates. Not only is the disease rate between the equator and latitudes 30 to 35 degrees north and south, but it becomes more common with increasing latitude thereafter. And yet, in Japan, regardless of its latitude, the disease is extremely rare. Another mysterious fact seems to be that if a person migrates from a high prevalence latitude to a warmer low prevalence latitude, he carries the high risk of MS (as the condition is frequently called) with him.

Though the condition doesn't follow *any* classical hereditary patterns, it is about eight times more common in immediate relatives (parents and siblings) than in the general population. This doesn't prove that it is hereditary, however; it may merely be a reflection of common exposure to an outside cause. (Thus, paralytic polio, which is certainly infectious and not hereditary, is also eight times more common in immediate family members than in the general population.)

It *is* known that in 2/3 of the cases the symptoms start between the ages of 20 and 40 and that there seems to be a slightly higher prevalence of the condition among women. Also, some recent studies have shown a shift toward its occurrence being more prevalent in higher socioeconomic groups than in the general population.

Again, though these do not prove causality, there are a number of known precipitating factors. MS may follow an acute infection of any type, various injuries, vaccinations, the injection of serum, or even during the course of a pregnancy. In some cases, emotional trauma seems to have been a precipitating factor.

Arising from this maze are two important *theories* of causation, one or both of which may very well prove to be correct. One theory is that a peculiar infection is acquired early in life—peculiar in that it has an extremely long incubation period and takes a long time to manifest itself. The other theory stresses the possibility of autoimmunity or special allergic reaction to one's own neurologic tissue.

So much for theories of causation. What is the disease itself like?

MS has a variety of complaints and findings, with remarkable periods of clearing followed by persistently recurring flare-ups. In about 40% of patients, the first symptom is one affecting the vision. There can be partial or total loss of vision in one eye, often associated with pain on movement of the eye—all of this occurring over just a few days. For those who are aware of the true fact that multiple sclerosis affects only the brain and not any part of the peripheral nervous system, it should be mentioned that the eye nerve is actually part of the brain. Within 2 weeks 1/3 of those afflicted with ocular symptoms will be on the road to complete visual recovery, 1/3 will have considerable improvement, and 1/3 will not improve. Incidentally, only about 40% of these 40% will ever go on to develop other manifestations of MS.

Some of these other manifestations include such nonspecific symptoms as tingling in the extremities, tight bandlike sensations around the trunk or limbs, double vision, transient loss of sensation of the face, dizziness, and vomiting. There may be actual weakness of the limbs and that peculiar kind of awkward stiffness known as spasticity of the limbs. There may be a peculiar way of speaking known as scanning speech in which the syllables of words are separated by prolonged pauses. There can be noticeable tremor of the head or arms and legs, and there can be incoordination of voluntary movements. Bladder symptoms of urgency, frequency, and even incontinence can occur. Impotence is not unusual. Convulsions, however, occur in only about 5%.

One of the most unusual of MS's symptoms is the peculiar euphoria or feeling of well-being that these patients have in the face of their obvious illness. This almost pathologic cheerfulness may be associated with apathy, lack of judgment, or inattention. Others, however, can be depressed, irritable, short-tempered, and may have memory losses.

Multiple sclerosis has one of the most peculiar courses in medicine. Some patients will have a series of flare-ups with varying combinations of the above symptoms, sometimes so severe that total paralysis and even coma may be present, followed by what seem to be complete remissions. Most patients will usually have, even during the periods of remission, some residual damage from the preceding flare-up, and each succeeding flare-up leaves further damage.

The actual duration of the disease is very variable. Though some patients may die in a few months, the average duration exceeds 20 years. At the end of 20 years, between 25% and 30% of patients are still actively carrying out their work.

There is no known cure for MS. ACTH (which is a pituitary hormone that stimulates the body's own cortisone-producing mechanisms) is used with some success in relieving symptoms in some patients and maybe even in decreasing the frequency of recurrences, but it does not cure the disease. In general, the patient should keep up with as much normal activity as he can, avoiding, however, overwork and fatigue.

TRANQUILIZERS AND SEDATIVES

"How tranquil can you get?" has been a disturbing question for the American medical community for over 10 years. The entire problem of tranquilizers and the freedom with which they are prescribed and dispensed has come under Federal Food and Drug Administration scrutiny.

The background to the "depressant and stimulant drug" investigation involves, in part, widely-publicized, flagrant violations of the existing laws and also much less heralded, though probably just as frequent, seemingly innocuous practices among many Americans. Among the former well-known and widespread infractions of the laws is that it's a rare community of 20,000 or more people which doesn't have its marijuana, pep pills, or addicting drugs problems. A problem with marijuana exists on every major college campus in the United States.

One example of the less publicized practices will illlustrate in how insidious a manner the abuse of such drugs can occur. A patient asked me if I could renew, for his wife, a prescription for a potent tranquilizer. After I explained that the writing of prescriptions was against our policy, I suggested he have the physician who originally ordered the drugs renew the prescription. He said that the physician was on the Pacific Coast since the drug had been ordered when they were living out there. On further inquiry, it turned out that his wife had not seen *any* doctor regarding this drug for over a year and was getting by on automatic prescription renewal. When I suggested that a new physician in this new home location might be needed to reevaluate the whole picture, the patient added that it didn't really make any difference what the doctor found because he, the patient's husband, knew his wife needed the drug! I even know of one patient who was having a prescription renewed which had been written by a physician who had long since died!

Some clarification of terms might be order. All addicting drugs are habit-forming, but not all habit-forming drugs are addicting. *Both* are important. Addiction to a drug involves the serious dependence upon a drug so that the patient's body requires its further administration to maintain normal physical and mental processes; upon the discontinuation of the drug, physical and mental derangements (the "withdrawal") occur. Addiction, therefore, involves a compulsion to continue the drug and obtain it by any means, a tendency to increase the dose, and the above mentioned physical-mental dependence. Heroin and morphine belong to this category (and their dispensing has long since been controlled by law). Alcohol also is a potentially addicting agent.

Habit-forming drugs involve a desire but not a compulsion to continue the drug, little or no tendency to increase the dose, some degree of psychic dependence ("habit"), but no physical dependence (no "withdrawal" or cessation). Among such drugs are "pep-pills," sedatives, and most tranquilizers.

In February 1966, a law covering the dispensing of such drugs as phenobarbital, seconal, nembutal, and the other barbituates, as well as benzedrine, dexedrine, and other pep pills went into effect. In May, 1966, the law was extended to include such widely prescribed drugs as Miltown (the most famous of the tranquilizers), Librium, Doriden (a non-barbituate sleeping compound), and six other depressants, as well as LSD, mescaline, and other drugs which have hallucinatory effects. Although these drugs have always been prescription items, prior to 1966, the writing of such prescriptions and dispensing of the drugs were not subject to any special handling or scrutiny.

The 1966 law required that there be no such thing as an "automatic refill" of such prescriptions. If a number of refills is designated by the physician, only that specified number will be honored so long as it is five times or fewer and so long as the refills are done within 6 months of the date of the original prescription. Telephone orders for such drugs will not be accepted.

The law further requires careful and extensive bookkeeping of all such transactions by physicians, pharmacists, drug manufacturers, and wholesalers. All such records are to be kept available for inspection for at least 2 years.

SLEEP

It has been estimated that there are millions of Americans who suffer sleep disorders of one form or another. The three chief manifestations are: (1) inability to get to sleep quickly upon retiring, (2) no trouble getting to sleep but waking up in the early morning hours (between 4 and 6 a.m.) and having little if any success in getting back to sleep thereafter, and (3) excessive sleepiness.

Before implying that each of the above conditions is always abnormal, we should realize that if a person is able to function normally, that is, carry out his normal routines of work and family life without being symptomatic (being too sleepy or exhausted to go on), then this may very well be a normal variant of human sleep patterns. While it is true that 7 or 8 hours of sleep are required for the majority of people, it is equally true that there is many a person who really seems to function well on little more than 4 or 5 hours sleep. These people usually are not overly tired during the day; while they may resort to an occasional week-end to "catch up" on missed sleep, this is not something they look forward to hungrily during the week. Equally normal are some people who just seem to need 9 or 10 hours of sleep. For them fewer hours results in the kind of exhausted tiredness and sleepiness that most of us feel when we haven't had a good night's sleep. A fairly good test of whether this is normal or abnormal is to find out how the patient feels about his sleep patterns and the performance of his daily activities.

Hypersomnia, which may be considered as the need to sleep more than 10 or 11 hours a day, is quite rare and probably deserves a thorough medical checkup to rule out such relatively rare diseases as brain tumors, underactive thyroid, severe kidney disease, and chemical poisoning. It has been suggested that the abnormal need for sleep in the absence of such medical problems may be an expression of a psychological problem in an attempt to "get away from it all" by seeking refuge in sleep.

Perhaps the most common of the sleep disorders is inability to fall asleep. These persons may spend up to 2 hours every evening tossing and turning before they can get to sleep. While it is possible that this may be due to such medical conditions as overactive thyroid, it is most often an expression of tension on the part of insomniacs. They often cannot "unwind" while the day's activities run through their minds or while they worry about what they are going to be doing the next day. Such persons while, naturally, are unhappy about losing sleep, nonetheless rarely prove to be suffering from a *major* psychological disorder.

The ones the physicians tend to be concerned about (because often the important psychological disorder called depression is the underlying cause of it) are the people who usually have no trouble falling asleep, but who wake up during the early morning hours and often just lie there, awake, until daybreak. Such a sleep pattern usually occurs in relatively brief periods of 2, 3, and 4 months rather than the often long-standing "inability to get to sleep" pattern.

There have been some interesting discoveries about sleep. Thus it has been learned that each night's sleep is composed of alternating cycles of a deep dreamless sleep and a much lighter dream-filled sleep. One of the remarkable findings from the sleep laboratories is that when subjects got 8 hours of dreamless sleep, they often awakened exhausted, while 4 to 5 hours of dream-filled, sometimes even bad dream-filled sleep, resulted in their awaking refreshed. These studies have emphasized, therefore, the importance of dreams, even though the person may not remember that he had been dreaming. Dreams seem to be an absolute prerequisite for a "good nights' sleep."

The reason this is important is that there are, again, millions of Americans who take some form of sleeping pill. How common it is to hear in doctors' offices someone exclaim, "I took my sleeping pill last night, I slept 7 solid hours, and I still feel utterly exhausted." Generally, in the past, physicians may have been tempted to attribute this to some neurotic dissatisfaction on the patient's part. We have now learned that while sleeping pills do make a person sleep, the overwhelming majority of sleeping pills result in dreamless sleep which the sleep laboratories have shown us is not a restful sleep. No wonder they were tired and exhausted in the morning!

This does not mean that no one should ever take a sleeping pill.

The acute agitation and excitement and sorrow at the death of a loved one or the serious illness of a family member may so upset a person that temporarily he may need a sleeping pill for a week or 10 days just to keep him from becoming ill from physical exhaustion. But for a person to take a sleeping pill regularly for months or years probably is depriving that person of the natural sleep which would have been better for him to obtain, even if it were in lesser quantities than he would obtain with a pill.

Another finding from the sleep laboratories is that after 3 or at most 4 weeks, most sleeping pills lose their effect until you switch to a different pill or raise the dose of the original pill. Since most doctors are very careful and cautious about increasing sleeping medications, we are left with millions of people who do take the same pill month after month in the same dose month after month, get the same dreamless sleep month after month, and continue to feel so tired and exhausted month after month that sleep and its problems become one of the big things of their days.

It is suggested that such patients see their doctors, who should be willing to spend all the necessary care and time to help wean them from their sleeping pill regimen. Insomnia very often is a conditioned reflex. Instead of expecting to drop to sleep as soon as they hit their pillow, that is often their signal for "the day and the week in review." Conditioned reflexes are hard to decondition but can be done; and if the patient is willing to "hold on" during the admittedly rough period of weaning away from sleeping pills and back to as normal a sleep as he could get, he may in the long run be grateful. He, in almost all cases, will be much better off for it.

DREAMS

We spend more than 30% of our lives asleep, and yet little is known about one important aspect of that period—dreaming. Recent work in the field has led us to modify our opinions so that dreams no longer are just a source of good stories to tell our friends or our psychiatrists but are being recognized as an important part of the physiological economy of the body.

To begin with, sleep is not a uniform state of unconsciousness; rather it is characterized by at least four levels of depth: Level 1, as shown by brain wave patterns, is closest to the waking state; and Level 4, furthest from the waking state. It is Level 1 that has come under close scrutiny recently. For one thing, it recurs four or five times during the course of an average night's sleep (its first appearance usually being not sooner than 50 to 90 minutes after the onset of sleep), it is associated with rapid eyeball movements (REM), and if you awaken a person during Stage 1 (REM stage), he almost always reports that he's been dreaming.

Contrary to what has been taught for years, dreaming does not take place in brief instances generally just before awakening; rather, it occurs throughout the night, in periods of varying length totalling up to 90 minutes in an average night's sleep, with an average of approximately 90 minutes between each REM cycle. And, it seems, just about everybody dreams; those who say they never dream just don't seem to remember their dreams.

One fascinating aspect of the dream or REM state is that young people spend more time in it than adults. Young children will spend 30–40% of their entire night's sleep in REM sleep; young adults, 20–25%, and older subjects, about 15%.

Besides rapid eye movements, Stage 1 sleep is associated with irregular, faster respirations (than Stage 4 sleep), an irregular, faster pulse rate, and increased variability in blood pressure. In short, the dream state resembles the active waking state even more than it does the quiet waking state, *e.g.*, lying in bed.

Perhaps the most intriguing of all the recent findings has been the discovery of how necessary the dream state is for all of us. For example, a group of volunteers was studied who were forcibly awakened every time their brain waves and other tests showed they were entering the REM stage. This went on for 5 nights in a row with a reduction of 80–90% of Stage 1 sleep. It was immediately noted that as time went on, more and more awakenings were required to keep the subjects from dreaming. During the first night four to five awakenings were enough; by the 5th night, 20–30 awakenings were required to keep the subjects from slipping into REM sleep. During the daytime the subjects were unusually tense and irritable, acting as though they had been deprived of a great deal of sleep even though they had actually slept 6–7 hours a night. On another occasion when these same subjects' sleep was interrupted for 5 nights during Stage 4 sleep, no daytime irritability was noted, nor was there so marked a day-by-day increase in the need for Stage 4 sleep.

Right after the 5 nights of REM sleep interruption, the subjects were allowed to sleep for 5 recovery nights without interruption. On such nights REM sleep was markedly increased, taking up to 30–40% of total sleep time; the subjects acted as if they were trying to "make up for" lost REM sleep.

Very recently subjects volunteered for up to 15 nights of REM-sleep (only) deprivation. It became so difficult to keep the subjects out of REM sleep along towards the 15th night that they had to be given dexedrine before retiring so that the experiment could continue. Recovery nights then showed up to 60% REM sleep! During the daytimes following REM-deprived sleep, not only were the subjects very irritable, but 2/3 of them showed distinct personality changes—some becoming quite paranoid, others becoming giggly and silly.

Some interesting facts have come to light regarding certain drugs and REM sleep. Phenobarbital, alchohol, and most of the other tranquilizers *decrease* the amount of REM sleep. Realizing the importance to the body's economy of this type of sleep, the question comes up of whether prolonged administration of transquilizers and sleeping pills *really* is a help to the patient or whether they might not contribute to his tension during the day. One group of researchers has proposed the theory that part of the reason chronic alcoholics suffer from hallucinations and "DT's" following sudden abstention from alcohol is that the body's continually increasing need for REM sleep becomes so great that it spills over into the waking state in the form of hallucinatory nightmarelike state we call DT's.

In general, it has been found that periods of increased stress during the daytime are associated with an increasing need for REM-stage sleep. It has been speculated that mental illness, with its concomitant increase in anxiety and disturbance, is usually associated with various degrees of inability to sleep, with its subsequent REM-sleep deprivation. At times, the dreams of the mentally disturbed are so frightening that they awaken him and thus deprive him further of REM sleep. Some of this deprivation then will spill over into the daytime symptoms of the severely disturbed, such as excessive fantasies and visual hallucinations which can therefore represent, on occasion, more the result of a superimposed REM-sleep deprivation than the underlying psychiatric problem. What is needed, and what medicine does not yet have, is a tranquilizer that will permit not only sleep, but also dreaming.

None of this is to say that in the wide spectrum of mental illness, lack of dreaming or disturbances of REM-type sleep are *causative* factors; rather such occurrences can at times aggravate the symptoms of emotional problems. Only under the experimental conditions of induced REM-sleep interruption and prevention can these occurrences be implicated as causative factors in daytime irritability and tension.

What about those who "never dream"? The new studies indicate that if interrupted right after REM-stage sleep, even these persons recall dreams. That they generally can't recall them is of no real significance. Certainly not being able to recall dreams is not a sign of not dreaming, nor is it in any way detrimental to the mental economy. Rather, it seems that nonrecallers are less introspective and less interested in the workings of their mind then are recallers—and such qualities may be more of a good than a bad thing!

13
Orthopedic

ARTHRITIS

Question: When is arthritis not arthritis?

Answer: When it is another basic disease, only one of whose manifestations is arthritis. To say about a joint problem, "This arthritis is caused by my getting older," may in most cases be true. However, in a significant minority of cases, other conditions can be present for which the treatment is essentially different from that of "run-of-the-mill" arthritis.

Osteoarthritis is not a real "disease" in the sense that rheumatoid arthritis is. It does not cause the fever, the weight loss, the anemia, and the changes in blood chemistries that are associated with a "systemic disease." It is a natural condition which occurs with increasing frequency as one gets older, affecting men and women equally (though it tends to occur a little earlier in men than in women, probably because men got more wear and tear on their joints at younger ages). By the time age 60 is reached, 97% of all people have some evidence of osteoarthritis.

Osteoarthritis is a disease of the joints, which is the result of the years of movements around them that occur as we age. It stays limited to the involved joints which will show little or no inflammation but which can be somewhat painful and may even, occasionally, develop some mild degrees of limitation of normal motion.

It generally begins as an aging destruction of the cartilage cushion at the ends of the joint bones. Eventually, bone may come to rest against bone, and as a result of their grating against each other, these may develop bone cysts, bone chips, and bone spurs. Since osteoarthritis *is* a condition of use and aging, the heavy weight-bearing joints are the ones most frequently involved: the hips, the knees, and the spine. Some nonweight bearing joints also frequently involved are the joints at the tips of the fingers and the joints at the base of the thumb and big toe.

The cause of osteoarthritis is obscure. Some persons (especially those who develop it relatively early in life) seem to be predisposed to it by heredity. In most, "wear and tear" and the amount of punishment a joint has to take seem to be the causative factors. That's why overweight people seem to be more susceptible to it and why a baseball pitcher is more likely to develop osteoarthritis in his throwing arm, especially his elbow.

Most people with osteoarthritis have no symptoms, even though there may be visible evidence of joint involvement. If there are symptoms, there are usually varying degrees of discomfort, ranging from mild aching and soreness, especially on movement, to pain which may even be present at rest. Another symptom is usually mild inability to perform easy, comfortable movements of the involved joint. Usually osteoarthritic joints are most painful after overuse.

What do you do if you have osteoarthritis? Nothing, if you're not having *real* symptoms of pain and limitation of motion. There is no cure for it so "catching it early" doesn't accomplish anything if it's not bothering you. If it *is* bothering you by pain then, depending on the severity and chronicity of the pain, there is medicine which can be taken for relief.

Plain old aspirin is probably the best drug that medicine has to offer for osteoarthritis. Because aspirin can be a very strong gastric irritant, take it at mealtimes or with an antacid. People tend to shrug off aspirin because it's so easily available and so widely used for so many conditions. They may not realize that for bone and joint afflictions, it is one of the best medicines *ever* discovered.

Aren't there other medicines? Phenylbutazone, indomethacin, and cortisone also work, BUT: (1) they are expensive and (2) they can be very dangerous. Not only can each one of these cause as much or even more gastric trouble than aspirin, but one or another of these can also (which aspirin does not do) cause destruction of the blood cells, abnormal retention of fluid in the body, a chemical hepatitis which can be fatal, skin rashes and other more serious forms of allergic reactions, kidney disease ranging from albumin in the urine all the way to kidney failure, high blood pressure and heart failure, neuritis of the eye nerves, hearing loss, high blood sugar, mental confusion, loss of hair, vaginal bleeding, and at times and especially in high doses, insanity. All this for a benign condition such as osteoarthritis? Aspirin, anyone?

Besides medications physical therapy can be valuable for osteoarthritis. It can help keep the joints flexible, help preserve the strength of muscles on which the joints depend for stability, and can help protect diseased joints against further damaging stresses. The necessary exercises aim at making sure the involved joints are moved through their full range of motion several times a day. Generally these are gentle and nonpainful rather than vigorous exercises.

Heat is another effective means of relaxing muscles and relieving pain and soreness in arthritic joints. Weight loss is another helpful thing in the overweight. There is, however, no such thing as an "arthritis diet" either to lose weight, help cure it, or stave it off.

In general, one has to learn to live with osteoarthritis. It is essentially a disease of aging even though no one ever died of it. If you have it and it's not bothering you at all, ignore it. If it's bothering you somewhat, ignore it if you can. If you *must* do something about it, consider aspirin, heat, physical therapy, and a good doctor.

Every other form of arthritis which is listed below is a manifestation not of a primary joint disease but of a systemic illness, some of whose major or minor manifestations appear in the joints.

An interesting fact that is often helpful in distinguishing osteoarthritis from the various other forms of arthritis listed below is that even though osteoarthritis is a primary affliction of the very joints themselves, quite often the external manifestations of the condition are less dramatic than in some of the conditions in which the arthritis is usually a secondary manifestation of a systemic disease.

Arthralgia is pain and discomfort in the joints without any external evidence of joint involvement. There is no redness, no swelling, no heat around the affected area. While it is unusual for the "systemic-joint" diseases to have only arthralgia, it is not at all uncommon for osteoarthritis to have arthralgia as its sole manifestation. Strictly speaking, arthritis, on the other hand, is arthralgia plus. Not only is the joint discomfort of arthralgia present in arthritis, but for it be classified as true arthritis, there should be some redness around the involved area or warmth greater than the surrounding tissues or at least some swelling. It is actually the exception rather than the rule, and an exception which is usually indicative of a relatively far advanced case, for there to be much, if any, redness or warmth around the osteoarthritic joint. There may be, however, swelling in such cases. We thus have the paradox of more external evidence of inflammation in conditions which secondarily affect the joints than in a disease which is primarily of the joints.

Second in frequency to osteoarthritis is rheumatoid arthritis. This is a chronic inflammation of the tough, fibrous connective tissue that holds parts of the body together. For no known medical reason, it strikes women between the ages of 18 and 45 three times as often as men of the same age.

The causes of rheumatoid arthritis are still cloaked in mystery. One long-standing theory is that an infection is responsible, but no germ has ever been isolated. Recently, however, significant studies have discovered suspicious tiny organisms in and around arthritic joints, some of them viruses, some bacteria, some not quite either. Other investigators lean to the theory that for some unexplained reason, the body's own defense mechanism breaks down. As a result, the body produces antibodies—substances that counteract the effects of invading organisms—which can begin to attack the body's own joints and tissues.

Rheumatoid arthritis comes on slowly. The first signs are a general tiredness, fever, loss of weight, and persistent joint soreness, stiffness, or swelling. Pain and stiffness are generally most severe on arising in the morning and lessen as the day goes on. The pain can disappear for months, then come on stronger than ever—and in more joints. Untreated, the joint could stiffen and twist as bone and cartilage erode. Bone ends can grow together so that they cannot be moved, making an arm or a leg useless. The surface of a joint can become so weak that it can no longer support a person's weight.

What can doctors do for victims of rheumatoid arthritis? They can prescribe a combination of drugs, exercises, and rest. Of all drugs, aspirin (in spite of the fact that it can cause severe gastric irritation) is still considered safest for long-term use by most arthritics. It relieves pain and reduces joint inflammation as well. Doctors generally prescribe much larger doses for arthritis victims than they would for cold or headache sufferers.

No matter which drug is used to treat arthritis, it is always used in combination with other methods of treatment. Special doctor-supervised exercises can help improve the function of the joints and keep the muscles strong. Heat from hot packs, electric pads, and lamps is often prescribed to relieve pain and inflammation. Splints and casts are used when necessary to prevent additional damage to an affected joint. In a number of cases, new types of orthopedic surgery have been successful in preventing deformities, increasing a joint's range of motion, and even replacing the entire hip joint.

Despite the availability of many legitimate sources of relief, shockingly large numbers of arthritis sufferers are being exploited today by promoters of worthless medications and useless devices. According to the Arthritis Foundation, victims of the disease spent $400 million last year on quack "cures," as opposed to only $15 million spent on legitimate arthritis research and training.

For example, new "wonder cures"—none new, nor a wonder, nor, of course, a cure—appear on the market almost every week. There are pills to take, liquids to drink, ointments to rub on, gases to breathe, and gadgets to wear, sit in, and be vibrated by. There are luxurious spas and clinics dispensing costly treatments "guaranteed" to end misery. Worst of all, there are some doctors who treat their arthritis patients with extremely powerful and dangerous drugs.

Modern drugs and other legitimate treatments can help most arthritis sufferers, but these valid treatments are not normally advertised in magazines, newspapers, or on radio or television. To find out about these remedies, people have to contact their doctor or the Arthritis Foundation.

The rest of the conditions in this article are also systemic conditions differing, however, from rheumatoid arthritis in the pattern of joint involvement. Thus, to have rheumatoid arthritis without joint involvement is almost a contradiction in terms. These other conditions can often be present without ever having joint involvement, but since the joints can be involved, it is always a good idea to see your doctor whenever a first or unusual attack of joint discomfort occurs.

Bacterial or other infections of various sorts can occasionally settle in a joint. Among the most common bacterial infections that can, on occasion, cause significant joint involvement are: gonorrhea, salmonella (the "food poisoning bacteria"), syphilis, and brucellosis. There is no distinguishing feature to these various arthritides that would help decide the diagnosis either one way or the other. They might very well present a picture of the garden variety of arthritis even though, in their cases, high dosages of antibiotics are usually mandatory in order to help control the infection before potentially dangerous joint destruction can occur.

BACK PROBLEMS

Pain in the back is, unfortunately, one of the most frequent of mankind's ills nowayears (that is, ever since he assumed the upright posture). The problem may range from just "a little stiffness when I wake up in the morning," all the way through various forms of arthritis, to the sometimes intractable disc problems which may require surgery.

Some of the causes of back symptoms seem mysterious and not at all obvious; for example, pain in the back can be secondary to a prostatic problem, or various diseases of the pancreas, or gall bladder disease, or peptic ulcer. But these causes (to be discussed later) are unusual, occur with other more specific symptoms, and really do not present a diagnostic problem to your doctor.

It's the structural back problems that are a pain. Briefly, the spinal column is a bony structure surrounding and protecting the spinal cord and the nerves that issue from it. In order to allow for such motions as twisting, turning, bending, etc., the spinal column is not one rigid single bone but rather is made up of a bunch of bones stacked up on each other, separated by a jellylike pulpy cushion called the intervertebral disc. This entire structure is enclosed by ligaments which help stabilize it while not interfering with its mobility. Further stabilization is provided by the large surrounding muscles whose contractions are responsible for our bending or moving in various directions.

The first question to be asked about an aching back is, "Where is the pain?" If the pain is in the upper part of the back, such conditions as a sprain of the rib muscles must be considered. Such discomfort is usually not in the midline but is either on one or the other side of the rib cage. The pain feels as if it were just slightly under the surface of the skin and is usually made worse by various movements which further increase the strain on the involved muscles.

Rarely, "back of the thorax" upper back pain is caused by a broken rib. In such cases the pain is usually in a very small localized area, directly over the broken bone. Also there is usually a very specific, obvious history of injury. Sometimes, the broken rib rubs over the lung lining (called the pleura), and it can irritate it so that the patient will experience sharp pain on breathing.

This leads to another of the upper back causes of pain—pleurisy. Years ago, when pneumonia was much more common, pleurisy was seen often because the infection deep in the lungs often inflamed the outer lung lining. The hallmark of pleurisy is pain on breathing or coughing. While a strained muscle or broken rib is a local condition, pleurisy is usually a sign of a more generalized, systemic type of illness, only one of whose problems is the pleurisy it causes.

Pain in the mid-back shifts the scene to other internal organs altogether. The mid-back is rather vaguely defined as the area between the bottom of the rib cage and the upper level of the hip bone. Here the most common cause of pain is sprain or spasm of muscle. Again, as in the case of rib cage muscle involvements, the pain will usually have followed either some prolonged or some unusual form of exertion.

A very, very excruciating, often cramping form of mid-back pain is the pain that accompanies the passage of a kidney stone. At times, infections of the kidneys themselves can cause a dull, chronic mid-back pain, but this is more a form of discomfort and is not in the same league as the pain of passing a kidney stone.

Other internal organs that can cause back pain are rare inflammation of the pancreas, serious uncontrolled peptic ulcers which are boring their way out of the duodenum onto the inner back muscles and thus causing them to go into spasm, and pain that is referred to the back from gallbladder disease. Gallbladder pain can be caused either by a severe infection of the gallbladder or by the passage of gallstones. Such pain, like kidney stone pain, is usually quite severe and cramping. Also like kidney stone pain, it is restricted to one side; in the case of gallbladder pain, this is almost invariably right-sided pain, either directly under the lower right rib cage area or, sometimes, extending right up to the rib cage area itself (which would then shift this to an "upper back" type of pain).

We now come to the low back which is where the pain usually is when people complain of their "aching back." "Lumbago," as such pain is often called, is not any specific condition itself but is just a not-so-fancy name for pain in the back. This is the area where diagnosis is difficult and treatment is, unfortunately, not always 100% satisfactory.

The three chief areas of problems that can cause low back problems are muscles, bones and joints, and, indirectly, nerves.

The great majority of low back pains are due to muscle strains: for example, a muscle which has not been regularly used and now has been overused in a short period of time or a normally used muscle which was twisted in a peculiar fashion so that a form of "charley horse" is afflicting it. Such muscular causes for low backs usually clear up within a week or 10 days at most. Often, no therapy is required. Aspirin, however, is an excellent medication for relief of muscle strain. Adding some dry heat in the form of a heating pad or a heating lamp might help further to speed up the recovery process.

Some persons are especially prone to muscular strains of the low back because of various bony asymmetries of their pelvis, unevenness of their hip line, curvature of the spine, etc. In such cases, your doctor can usually advise you as to which motions are especially to be avoided.

A second and much less frequent cause of low back pain is due to a problem with the bone structure itself. Usually, the sacrum (which is the bone in the low back that unites the two hip bones) will have some changes of arthritis. Often, such arthritic changes will be visible on X-ray, but this is not so in the early stages, so a negative X-ray doesn't mean that arthritis is absolutely out of the question.

There are two forms of arthritis that can involve the low back. The common one is osteoarthritis which generally afflicts older persons, usually well over the age of 50 and, though not a crippling form of arthritis, can nonetheless cause enough discomfort that your doctor might very well recommend medication to relieve the inflammation. Once again, perhaps the best medicine of all is aspirin.

A rare, but nonetheless, serious form of bone back problem due to arthritis is that caused by rheumatoid arthritis. Rheumatoid arthritis of the low spine occurs more often in men than in women, usually at a relatively young age (in the 20's). While it does respond to aspirin, this often is a progressive and serious condition of the entire body and requires regular examinations and follow-up by a competent specialist in rheumatoid arthritis problems. Any recurrent low back pain in a young man that often has nothing to do with exertion and doesn't resemble a kidney problem at all should be thoroughly evaluated for the possibility of rheumatoid arthritis.

A final cause of low back problems is nerve pressure. This is the one most people know about even though it is not common. This is the true "sciatica." It is caused by partial or complete rupture of the ligaments that hold the cushioning material between the lower spinal vertebrae. This results in a partial or complete extrusion of this cushioning material from between the vertebrae. Since the branches of the sciatica nerve also pass out through this small opening between the vertebrae, this cushioning, "disc" material presses upon the nearby nerve. The sciatic nerve which goes down the buttocks to the legs is one of the longest, largest and most vulnerable nerves in the body. Sciatica pain is distinguished by a pain which is usually very specific in its localization. Not only is it pain in the back, but it is also pain down the back of the buttocks and thigh, and sometimes even down the back of the calf. Often there is numbness, and not infrequently the person is in such acute pain he can barely stand up and get about.

Obviously, taking aspirin is not going to make the ruptured disc go back into place. This particular problem, if it doesn't clear up itself in a week or so, often requires hospitalization with traction. Such traction, by putting weights on the bottom part of the body, attempts to stretch the distances between the vertebrae so that, hopefully, the ruptured disc will pop back in. If this is not successful, surgery is often required because true sciatic pressure, if left untreated, can cause permanent damage to the muscles of the leg.

Once an acute problem has subsided there are some things a person "with a weak back" should remember. Generally persons with back problems should not do too much standing; when they are standing or walking they should walk with feet straight ahead, letting most of their weight come down on their heels rather than the balls of their feet. This is why women with back problems are usually advised not to wear high-heeled shoes. When walking, one should walk with one's chest up and out because this helps to settle the weight on the heels.

Many persons have the idea that it's good for the back, when sitting, to sit stiffly upright with shoulders thrust back militarily, thus emphasizing the curve in one's back. This is wrong. As a matter of fact, persons with back problems are urged to learn to live as if they did not have a hollow in their back—when sitting, standing, or walking.

When sitting they are urged to sit, if possible, with their knees higher than their hips (thus helping to eradicate the hollow in the back). Even when they are sleeping, they are urged to sleep with one or both knees drawn up, whether they sleep on their backs or their sides. (Incidentally, beds of people with back problems should be firm.) When standing they are urged not to bend backwards because this would accentuate the hollow of their backs (which is to be avoided).

Finally, such persons are advised to pay special attention to the way they lift things. They should always squat when lifting, never bending forward to lift with knees straight. Also, when they do straighten up with the lifted object, they should not lift it above the waist line, for in doing so they will be arching back the upper part of their body, and this will bring out the hollow in their back. While they lift, they should carry the load close to the body, keeping the back as straight as possible. They are urged to lift with their arm and leg muscles, not their back muscles.

BACK EXERCISES

The exercises that will be covered here are good exercises to help strengthen your low back muscles and thus should be helpful in preventing the most common cause of back discomfort: muscle strains. It should be emphasized, however, that strengthening your back muscles will not in any way relieve the back problems that are due to the two other leading causes that we mentioned in the previous article: various forms of arthritis and sciatic nerve pressure. As a matter of fact, anyone for whom the diagnosis of true sciatica has been raised should not undertake any program of exercise, including the one mentioned here, without first consulting with his own physician and getting a specific program of exercises that is tailored to his needs.

Modern man's daily existence is unfortunately largely composed of sedentary living, often on his job and usually combined with a lack of any significant recreational exercise. The resultant loss of muscle tone leaves the back vulnerable to the sudden stress that will occur following unusual heavy exertion. Actually, even poor muscle tone in one's abdominal area (and who among us doesn't suffer from that!) can result in chronic muscle imbalance that further stresses the low back.

The following list of exercises should not take up much time; but it is important that they be performed regularly, at least three or four times a week, and from here on out. Period! You can't exercise for 3 or 4 years only and expect that that should take care of your back for the rest of your life. Regular exercise is a valuable help in strengthening the muscles so long as you continue to do it.

Many a person has trouble flexing his trunk forward because of a tight low back. A good stretching exercise for this can be accomplished by lying on your back and alternately pulling both knees to your chest. If performing this results in no discomfort, one can then go on to bringing both knees simultaneously to touch the chest. This "knee hug" exercise should be held for at least 30 seconds, if possible, followed by a gradual release.

Weak abdominal muscles can be strengthened by the following exercise which is an especially good one because it can be executed without strain being placed on the low back. To perform the "abdominal curl," lie on your back with your knees bent and your feet on the floor. Maintain the knees in this fully flexed position, bring your chin to your chest, and slowly curl the trunk upward as though you were going to touch your forehead to your knees, keeping the chin on the chest all the time. In performing this exercise, the hands and arms should not be hugging the knees; rather they should be kept parallel to the floor as the upper part of your trunk gradually lifts itself. You will not be able to come up far enough to touch the forehead to the knees; however, the exercise should be as if you were going to do that.

A good muscle stretcher for the entire body, including the low back, is this one: lie flat on the floor with the arms fully extended upward so that the hands are pointing completely in the opposite direction from your feet. The back of your hands should be touching the floor. Extend the arms all the way up and reach as far back as possible, stretching at the same time so that your toes point as far down from your body as possible. Don't arch the back. Then, relax the right leg and the left arm and stretch crosswise so that the left heel and the right hand are at maximum distance apart. Repeat this with the opposite arm and leg, always remembering to relax completely after each stretch. This exercise can also be done four or five times.

A final exercise that I would suggest you do in absolute privacy (because you will look silly if you do it with anyone watching you) is called the "mad cat" exercise. Starting in an all-fours position, let the weight on your body rest on your hands and knees, then arch your low back by tightening the stomach and buttock muscles as you inhale. Anyone looking at you will see that you do indeed resemble an angry cat. Then, lean forward, keeping the back arched, by bending the arms until the forehead touches the floor, exhale, and return to the starting position.

As a final reminder of some good things to do for your back: don't sit too long; getting up and walking around your desk is not only good for your back but also is good for the circulation of your lower extremities. Finally, and this is the hardest of all, try to avoid tension because chronic muscular tension is certainly a contributor to low back pain.

BURSITIS

Is there ever anyone who reaches, say, age 65 without experiencing, at least once in his lifetime, an attack of bursitis? I'm beginning to doubt it, especially because there are 140 or more bursae in the human body, and bursitis often seems to be just a natural concomitant of aging.

A bursa is a closed, fluid-filled sac that is found in many places in the body. Basically the fluid in the bursa serves as a cushioning agent which helps to facilitate the play of one structure of the body over another. There are only a few drops of lubricant fluid in most bursae since most of them are quite small. The walls of the bursa are extremely smooth and ride on each other with a minimum of friction. Some bursae are found directly under the skin, between it and underlying bony prominences such as the elbow and the knee. Other bursae are placed under the thin fibrous sheets of tissue into which muscles often taper. The presence of these bursae allow the tissue sheets to ride over underlying structures such as bones with a minimum of friction and, thus, no discomfort. Some bursae serve to cushion one tendon from another or a tendon from underlying bone.

Most bursae are present at birth, but some develop later on in response to repeated friction. Some of the more superficially placed bursae (usually the ones between bony prominences and skin) are not essential for function and can actually be destroyed or removed with no significant loss in function. Other deeper bursae (those situated between bony prominences and muscle or tendon, or around joints) are quite important to the body; and treatment of bursitis in these structures usually must aim toward preservation of the basic bursa.

Some of the greatest descriptive names in all of medicine are associated with some of the more common types of bursitis. The only one lacking such a fanciful title happens to be the most common of all bursites: the shoulder bursitis that causes the painful shoulder that so many people think is the *only* form of bursitis. Perhaps next in frequency is "tennis elbow" which is merely a bursitis around the elbow and quite often occurs in people who've never held a tennis racket in their lives. Then we have "soldier's heel" which is a bursitis at the back of the heel. (There is even a relatively common bursitis on the bottom part of the heel which, so far, doesn't have any fancy title.)

Another titleless bursitis that is quite common occurs over the bony protuberance at the upper outer part of the thigh. This trochanteric bursitis is especially painful when one tries to rotate the hip outwardly. The common bunion of the foot is a bursitis which usually overlies a prominent misshapen curvature where the big toe joins the rest of the foot.

One of the great names in medicine is "weaver's bottom" which is probably self-explanatory: presumably caused by the hard surfaces the weavers used to sit on for hours as they plied their trade, weaving back and forth on their bottoms. And how many of us have gone through life without realizing that "nun's knee" was the same as "rug cutter's knee" and that both were the same as "housemaid's knee." And then there's "miner's elbow."

There is, however, one thing that all bursites have in common: pain. Since a bursitis is really the same condition, basically, regardless of where it occurs, what will follow now applies to all bursites, regardless of location. There are two chief forms of bursitis—acute and chronic. Acute bursitis has pain in the inflamed bursa with localized swelling and tenderness which is usually due to the accumulation of various inflammatory fluids into the involved bursal sac. One of the hallmarks of an acute bursitis is limitation of motion around the involved area. Sometimes the inflammation is so acute that even the weight of clothing over the involved area is painful to the patient. In most cases, the inflammatory exudate is absorbed by the lining cells of the bursa, and the acute attack is over within a week or two. However, the condition may become chronic.

Acute bursitis may be caused by any of a number of factors, the chief of which is probably unknown. Single or repeated trauma (remember the praying nun or the shuttling weaver) is often blamed and may indeed be a factor, but as mentioned above, there's many a case of tennis elbow that occurs in non-tennis players; often it will occur in the arm that a person doesn't usually use. Even rarer causes of acute bursitis include gout, acute or chronic infections, and at times rheumatoid arthritis.

Chronic bursitis is the other chief form of bursitis. It usually follows previous episode(s) of acute bursitis or repeated trauma or may be due to chronic foci of infection. Again, often, it just occurs with no clearly discernible cause. In contrast to acute bursitis which tends to hurt spontaneously, chronic bursitis' pain usually follows unusual exercise or effort. There may or may not be swelling due to underlying fluid accumulation; but there is always limitation of motion, especially in certain specific positions of the structures around the involved bursae. Chronic bursitis may last from a few days up to months.

What does one do for bursitis? For acute bursitis, complete rest of the involved part is a must during the early stages of exquisite pain. Sometimes it's even necessary to put the part (*e.g.,* an arm in shoulder bursitis) in a sling or splint it or rest it on a pillow or other support. Such dramatic restrictions are necessary only until the pain and the surrounding localized muscle spasm begin to subside. For those who "need something" for the pain, aspirin, with or without the addition of a narcotic pain killer, is usually sufficient. Some doctors recommend local heat applications in the form of compresses or an electric pad, even though one's initial impression would be to use cold. In those unusual circumstances in which the application of heat seems to aggravate the pain, ice packs may help. Massage, diathermy, or ultrasonic treatments are also helpful for acute bursitis.

In order to avoid the unfortunate complication of adhesive bursitis or "frozen joint," it is recommended that active movements be undertaken as soon as the pain begins to come under control. If the acute pain episode seems to be unusually persistent, the injection of a local anesthetic or a cortisone compound is sometimes used. Sometimes fluid is aspirated from the acute joint before the medications are instilled—and, at times, this aspiration of fluid may have to be repeated once or twice.

On very rare occasions where pain persists for more than a week, X-ray treatments have usually been successful. It is only if X-ray treatments prove unsuccessful in particularly stubborn cases of bursitis that surgical intervention is resorted to.

What does one do for chronic bursitis? Diathermy, hot packs or baths, even massage may help—temporarily. Cortisone injections have proved helpful. Sometimes it is necessary to break up the calcium that is often deposited in a chronic bursitis by needling it under anesthesia or during a cortisone injection. Exercises to correct or prevent surrounding muscle wasting are always in order.

14
Respiratory

EMPHYSEMA

"Doc, what's all this I keep hearing about emphysema nowadays? You never used to hear about it 25 or 30 years ago. Have you people invented a new disease or something?"

The patient that spoke thus to me had grasped some of the truth; while it isn't true that doctors have recently invented emphysema, it *is* true that the condition is much more prevalent now than it was 30 or so years ago. And, from the way cigarette smoking continues to increase in our population, emphysema promises to be even more prevalent in the future than it is now.

In order to understand just what emphysema is, we must keep in mind the primary function of the lungs which is to get oxygen into the blood and to remove gaseous waste products, especially carbon dioxide, out of the blood. To accomplish this the lungs act like a big bellows. When we inhale, the bellows expands and air (containing oxygen) rushes from the back of the throat down the lung tubes (called bronchi) all the way to the many small air sacs, where it comes into contact with the minute blood vessels of the lung. It is at this level that the vital exchange occurs. Oxygen enters the blood vessels and carbon dioxide leaves them. Now exhalation begins; the bellows collapse and the gaseous contents rush back up and out of the lungs.

Basically, in emphysema, the bellows action is lost. The lungs have become so stiff and distended from chronic irritation or chronic infection that their normal pliability is gone. The collapsing of the bellows that is normal exhalation becomes very difficult, if not impossible; as a result carbon dioxide and other waste gases that should be exhaled accumulate in the lungs and back up in the blood.

Furthermore, although the lungs are relatively fixed in the open bellows position, inspiration also becomes difficult in emphysema because getting air in involves the opening of a previously closed bellows. A bellows fixed in an open position really can't open much more, and so people with emphysema have trouble getting oxygen into their lungs.

A further factor that often complicates the loss of elasticity of the lungs is spasm of the walls of the bronchi leading down to the air sacs. Naturally, a narrowed tube allows for the passage of less air than if it were open.

Ultimately, as the above picture progresses, normal breathing which should be automatic, easy, and unrestricted is lost, to be replaced by wheezing and chronic cough, at first dry but eventually productive of phlegm, especially in the mornings. Shortness of breath is present, mild at first, but eventually progressing to the point where the slightest exertion (such as putting on one's shoes) will leave the patient blue and literally gasping for air. Soon breathing itself becomes hard work and is, in turn, exhausting so that finally one is left with a pulmonary cripple for whom breathing is a desperate, painful struggle for air. Eventually they can go on and die of suffocation.

What's the cause of this truly horrible disease? Chronic bronchitis is an important cause and may be a combination of chronic irritation as well as chronic infection. Recent studies have cast very strong suspicion upon smoking as one of the chief factors in the causation of emphysema—and statistics indicate that as smoking has increased throughout our population so has the frequency of emphysema. That's why one is beginning to see women now with the condition where previously it had been seen almost exclusively in men. It takes 20 years or so of smoking to cause the damage. As we begin to have an increasing number of women with this much smoking behind them, we are learning that emphysema is not a respecter of sex.

What can be done about emphysema? To begin with, one point must be made clear: It is an irreversible condition. One can never return to a normal lung; *but* one can keep the condition from progressing by avoiding the incriminated chronic irritants, especially smoking, and by treating vigorously all lung infections by antibiotics and various measures of sputum drainage. There are also drugs available to relieve spasm of the lung tubes. Finally there are breathing exercises the patient can do to help increase the efficiency of whatever bellows action is left.

That doesn't sound like much one can do, but it's all that doctors have to offer nowadays. That's why so much emphasis must be placed on prevention. In this case an ounce of prevention (such as stopping smoking) is worth more than a pound of cure, since there is no cure.

RESPIRATORY ILLNESS

It may very well be true that people get more respiratory infections in the winter than at any other season of the year, ranging all the way from the common cold up to pneumonia. Luckily for everyone concerned, the progression from the former to the latter is not inevitable. The chief respiratory illnesses that afflict people are: the common cold, bronchitis, sinusitis, pneumonia, and influenza, each of which has enough considerably distinct symptoms that one can usually be readily distinguished from another.

By far the most common of these infections is the common cold. The common cold is always caused by a virus, but the likelihood of one's getting it doesn't depend so much upon one's exposure to that virus as it does upon one's inherent susceptibility. When you have a high resistance against that particular virus infection, then all the exposure to it is not going to cause you to get a common cold. The hallmark of the common cold is that the symptoms are restricted to what is called the upper respiratory passages. There will be nasal congestion and a significant runny nose. There will be a raspy throat. There may even be loss of one's voice. One's ears may get clogged. One's sinuses may clog. One may get sinus headache. One often gets a low grade fever, usually well below 100 degrees. The cold seems to travel from one area to another—the nose, the sinuses, the throat—and then in 7 or 10 days it is all gone. No antibiotics are needed because this is a pure virus infection.

The common cold usually doesn't have much, if any, cough. If coughing is present, then in most cases the common cold has progressed to bronchitis. Most bronchitis is also a virus affliction, and most bronchitis is usually preceded by an upper respiratory common cold. So, the typical picture of bronchitis is that added to all the above symptoms, one develops after about the first 5 or 6 days a deep cough, at first a dry hacking cough, which can be so annoying that it actually keeps one from sleeping well. There is also often an associated burning sensation under the breastbone. After 2 or 3 days of this dry cough, phlegm and mucus are produced, at first throughout the day, but then usually mainly in the morning shortly after arising. Because bronchitis is a more extensive involvement of the respiratory tract, there often is more temperature elevation than in the common cold. However, with an uncomplicated viral bronchitis, the temperature usually doesn't go above 101 degrees, and the material that is brought up from the lungs is generally whitish. The presence of thick, greenish or yellowish sputum or of blood-streaked sputum is most unusual for bronchitis and makes one think of one of two possibilities—either the bronchitis has turned into a bacterial bronchitis or the person has developed pneumonia. While the usual cough with bronchitis doesn't require antibiotics because of its viral nature, a bacterial super-infection causing the thickened, discolored sputum and fever of at least 101 degrees usually requires the administration of antibiotics for 4 or 5 days until the temperature has been normal for at least 24 hours.

The only other relatively common complication of an acute cold which would require the administration of antibiotics would be the development of what is called a purulent sinusitis. While the sinus involvement of a cold results in the production of copious whitish mucus, a purulent sinusitis is associated with significantly discolored mucus: yellowish, greenish discharge and some more temperature elevation than one would have with an uncomplicated common cold. Both viral sinusitis and bacterial sinusitis would each have sinus congestion and pain and headache over the involved areas, so one cannot use these symptoms to distinguish between the two of them. The character of the mucus is what really is the clue. As in the case of bacterial bronchitis, antibiotics are indicated for bacterial sinusitis.

Pneumonia is a different and more serious animal altogether, and we are not really sure why it is much less common than it used to be 30 or 40 years ago. While it is true that some pneumonias can be caused by viruses, it is generally the case that pneumonias are bacterial infections requiring vigorous and prompt antibiotic administration. How often do we see a case of a common cold progressing to a sinus infection, then bronchitis, then pneumonia? Rarely—except in people who have some kind of chronic disease which is lowering their resistance to all infections in general. Not at all uncommon for the person who has pneumonia is for them to develop in a day or so at most, almost out of the clear blue sky, a lot of deep cough, a significant amount of fever (usually 102 degrees or more), pain in one side or other of the chest, not only on coughing and deep breathing but sometimes even on shallow breathing, and also the production of discolored, thick sputum, often tinged with blood flecks. While pneumonia is not considered an absolute medical emergency, it still is a very serious illness requiring prompt medical attention.

Often associated with pneumonia is a condition called pleurisy. Pleurisy is an inflammatory involvement of the outer lining of the lung so that when the lung rubs against the chest wall, the protective lining hurts because it is inflamed. As the underlying infection, usually pneumonia, subsides, the pleurisy resolves itself also. Rarely, if ever, is pleurisy a primary disease in itself, but rather it is a symptom and sign of an underlying problem.

There are few true viral pneumonias that are caused by the same virus that causes common colds or bronchitis. They are usually the result instead of an atypical organism which, luckily, is often susceptible to antibiotics. This is a decision that has to be made by your own doctor at the time of examination. At times viral pneumonia has a very special type of picture on X-ray differing from the usual X-ray abnormality of the typical bacterial pneumonia. (Bronchitis, as well as the common cold, present a completely normal chest X-ray.)

Finally, influenza: influenza is a virus disease that is diagnosed as such much more often than it is truly present. The influenza virus is not the cause of the common cold, and true influenza causes a sort of combination of symptoms from the above-described diseases. Though the upper respiratory tract is involved, the thick nasal and sinus congestion and the clogged ears of a common cold are lacking, but there may be some sore throat. It has the dry cough aspects of bronchitis but is usually lacking the mucus production of bronchitis. It has the generalized feeling of ill-being and body aches of a major infection, such as pneumonia; but except in those who are very weak and rundown, it is not so serious as pneumonia. Added to it are severe muscle discomforts, especially in the low back and calves. Many people complain of nagging discomfort in the eyes; even moving the eyes back and forth causes discomfort. Again, since this is a virus infection, antibiotics are not indicated. However, since it is such a relatively wide-ranging infection, it tends to lower one's resistance—considerably lower than in the case of a common cold or even a common cold complicated by bronchitis, so that in more than a few cases the susceptibility to a bacterial pneumonia is significantly increased in people who have had a true attack of influenza. This is why recovery is prolonged and why careful attention should be given to patients during such attacks.

EFFECT OF SMOKING ON OTHERS

A reader of my column once wrote me an interesting letter from which I quote the following paragraph:

For some months, I have been working closely with a man who constantly smokes a pipe. His smoke fills the work area everyday. It is not just tobacco smoke which makes me nauseated but the way he makes use of his pipe and the manner he discards the tobacco ashes and uses pipe cleaners. By refilling tobacco, he smokes the same pipe for hours. The odor is atrocious and offending mainly because his saliva drips into his pipe bowl and incessant burning of the soggy tobacco. In addition, he discards the used pipe cleaners and burnt but soggy ashes in the nearby waste basket. Sometimes, it is hard to say whether the odor from the pipe is stronger than that of the waste basket.

The reader asked that I comment about this in a column. The reason I have quoted so extensively from his letter is that the answer to it must consider both aspects. (1) The considerable medical effects of the smoke upon nonsmokers, and (2) the social discomfort caused by some of the disgusting habits some smokers have. It may turn out that the latter problem, which is more a social one than a medical one, is more important than the former. While there are some unpleasant and perhaps even potentially harmful effects of smoke upon nonsmokers, I do not believe there is overwhelming medical evidence that would allow physicians to make the statement, "Inhalation of tobacco smoke by most well nonsmokers is dangerous to their health." However, with the increasing awareness of the danger of tobacco smoke to smokers themselves, many nonsmokers have become "gun shy" and more willing to speak up about the social discomfort inflicted upon them by the careless smoker. It may turn out to be that the appeal to common courtesy and decency and consideration for others will be more successful than citing some of the medical effects to the offended nonsmoker. After all, many is the smoker who has refused to give credence to the solid data of the U.S. Surgeon General and the medical profession regarding the absolute danger to his health of smoking; that such a person would alter his smoking habits for the benefit of another person, based on some medical facts which everyone admits are considerably weaker than those that apply to the smoker himself, is quite unlikely.

One known uncontroverted side effect of tobacco is that it is a definite irritant to a person's eyes and the mucous membranes of the upper respiratory tract. Everyone's eyes will be irritated, to a greater or lesser degree, by smoke in a room, whether it is one's own smoke or that of others. Of course, persons with sensitive eyes, either intrinsically or based on previous or chronic eye conditions, will be most afflicted by the particulate matter that makes up tobacco smoke. In a similar fashion, it is those persons who have a chronic respiratory problem, such as asthmatics, who will have the most irritation to their respiratory mucous membranes from the tobacco smoke.

The burning of tobacco results in the release into the surrounding area not only of irritants, such as just mentioned, but also of small amounts of chemicals that have been shown to cause cancer in animals. A study in *Preventive Medicine* indicated that there are substances released into the air which inhibit the beneficial cleansing motion of the little hair cells that line the respiratory tract. At high enough concentrations, such chemicals can actually prevent the normal "housecleaning" that our lungs do all day long to keep bacteria and other foreign substances from causing damage.

Another substance that results from the burning of tobacco is carbon monoxide which can rise, in the air surrounding smokers, to levels which are 1/3 that found in dense urban automobile traffic. Nicotine can be so absorbed from the polluted air that results from tobacco smoke that it can be found in the urine of nonsmokers. However, there aren't yet very significant data available to demonstrate any really adverse health effects from the nicotine levels reached in adult nonsmokers, and the carbon monoxide concentrations in nonsmokers are far below levels that are known to be hazardous to health.

It may be, however, that the studies are of too brief a duration and too recent an onset. Perhaps, in a few years, more significant data will be available. One interesting study, that might be an indication of something like this, showed that there is an increased prevalence of acute respiratory disease in young children whose parents smoke.

We may best sum up the medical significance of smoking on nonsmokers by quoting Dr. David M. Burns, formerly the federal government's top medical man on the smoking and health issue, "There is ample evidence that involuntary smoking causes annoyance and minor eye and throat irritations to a substantial percentage of the population. It may cause major and, occasionally, life threatening problems to people with heart and lung disease." On the other hand, a very good point regarding the social offensiveness of tobacco smoking was made by the well-known epidemiologist, Dr. James P. Dunn, when he wrote: "I do not believe, for example, that employees would be allowed to burn incense or play radios or tape recorders if these proved to be annoying to other workers. I believe every effort should be made to restrict smoking where possible and, in office areas, to consider rearrangement of individuals to reduce the annoyance factor as low as possible." To both of these statements I append a fervent "Amen."

15
Miscellaneous

AEROTITIS

Good hearing is something many of us take for granted, and as a result we sometimes don't take as much care of our ears and hearing as we should. We all expect that our hearing, along with our eyesight, will decrease in range along with the aging process; and we know that much of this decline is inevitable. Illnesses or accidents can, however, markedly accelerate this hearing loss. They are treatable or avoidable if only we'd follow some elementary rules.

There is a canal from the outer ear in to the ear drum which is called the external auditory canal. This is the passage where wax accumulates and where children like to store small foreign objects. Behind the ear drum is the middle ear, where the three ear bones transmit the sound from the ear drum to the inner ear or cochlea. The middle ear has the Eustachian tube opening out of it and leading down to the back of the throat. It's because of this passage that we hear the click of the equalization of pressure on both sides of the ear drum when we yawn or move our jaw in special ways.

The inner ear is a bone-encased circular set-up on which the middle ear bones terminate in the transmission of sound. This fluid-filled inner ear structure not only serves for hearing but also serves as one of the organs which helps us maintain our balance. From the inner ear there are two nerves (which are really an extension of the brain and not part of the ear itself) which carry the hearing and balance sensations to selective portions of the brain.

The increase in air traveling has brought to the fore a condition called aerotitis. This can prove to be not only troublesome and painful, but it can also lead to permanent damage to one's hearing. Basically what happens in such cases is that the person has a head cold with all the nasal, sinus, and throat congestion that goes along with it. Often the throat side of the opening of the Eustachian tube also becomes swollen, or the tube itself can become congested.

As a result, the free passage of air up and down the tube becomes obstructed, leading to a complete or partial loss of the ability to equalize the pressure on both sides of the ear drum. When one isn't going from one different pressure level to another, this isn't too serious a problem.

However, when one does go to different pressure levels, as in flying, this can prove to be a real problem. When one goes up in a plane, the pressure in the outer ear goes down. Meanwhile, the pressure in the middle ear (which has a congested blocked Eustachian tube exit) remains unchanged at a higher level than in the outer ear. In most cases, the middle ear pressure continues to build up, so that finally it can force some of its way out through the swollen Eustachian tube. Equal pressure in the middle and outer ear results.

The situation, unfortunately, is different when one begins the descent. Now the pressure in the outer ear begins to rise, but the middle ear pressure remains relatively lower. In this case, the blocked Eustachian tube acts like a one-way valve: it will let an increased air pressure leak out from the middle ear down to the throat, but it will not generally let an increased air pressure in the throat go up to the middle ear. Consequently, a relative vacuum results in the middle ear.

In mild cases, the person will experience stuffiness of the ears on descent which is not relieved by yawning. The ear drum will retract inwards, pushed by higher air pressure in the outer ear. Since the bones that transmit sound through the middle ear are attached directly to the ear drums, hearing also is affected.

In more severe cases, the person may suffer excruciating pain, and hemorrhages may occur in the middle ear behind the ear drum. Because pressure equalization can't take place through the blocked Eustachian tube, the middle ear fills up with the bloody fluid from its own lining to help keep the ear drum from exploding inwards toward the relative vacuum created by the descent to the higher air pressure areas.

Many of these people have symptoms that clear in a day or two, but the condition may last for 1 to 3 weeks.

What should be done about all this: prevention. In mild colds a doctor should be consulted to see if there are medicines he can give to help shrink the congested Eustachian tube membranes before going on a flight. If this is not successful, don't fly. Do not fly when you have a moderate or severe upper respiratory infection. Those who have experienced such discomfort on flights should contact a doctor right away.

HEIMLICH MANEUVER

Death by choking on food has become widely pubicized as a "cafe coronary." Aside from the fact that "cafe coronary" is a catchy title, another reason it is an apt designation for the condition is that it summarizes the usual conditions under which such accidents occur: People in cafes usually not only eat but also drink, and it has been postulated that were the various swallowing and choking reflexes of the back of one's throat not dulled by the previous ingestion of often significant amounts of alcohol, the choking episode would probably never have occurred in the first place. While there is much truth in the theory that ingestion of alcohol can be a factor, nonetheless I have been personally present where alcohol was not involved at all; so, we must not be fooled into thinking that this only occurs in drunken old people whose false teeth fit so loosely that they can't chew food well enough, causing them to choke on a large piece of food. And that is the significant factor—the large morsel of food. This, however, is the *sine qua non* of the condition: Unlike alcohol which may or may not be present, if there is no large chunk of unchewed food, "cafe coronaries" don't occur. One of the original horror stories in relation to this condition tells of a person choking on an unchewed piece of steak that was as large as a pack of cigarettes!

What happens in such a case is that this large morsel "goes down the wrong way," entering the trachea or windpipe rather than the esophagus or gullet. In those cases in which the piece is too big to enter the windpipe, it often lies on top of the opening, effectively blocking it off. As a person tries to gasp at the occurrence, this only pulls the material tighter against the windpipe since gasping is really taking in a deep breath of air. Since this thing is sitting on top of the windpipe, when you try to take in a deep breath, all you manage to do is pull it more tightly shut against the opening.

One of the hallmarks of a "cafe coronary" is the silence surrounding it. When a person makes a sound, be it speech, or a cough, or a cry, what he is doing is utilizing the air that is passing back and forth over his vocal chords. The trouble with a "cafe coronary" is that no air is passing back and forth anywhere, and so the person cannot make any sound; thus one often sees a redfaced, silent victim who is obviously in great distress. The one case I was present at involved a person at dinner who suddenly got up, very redfaced, literally ran around the room once and then out of the room, all without uttering a sound, to the astonishment of the onlookers. When he was in the other room, he treated his own "cafe coronary" by reaching into the back of his throat and plucking out the offending morsel. That was followed by one of the loudest gasping whoops I have ever heard.

And that essentially was what originally brought this condition to medical attention. Here was an accident that could be fatal in 5 or 6 minutes if nothing was done, and yet the cure was as simple as reaching into the back of the person's throat and plucking out the offending agent with the middle and index fingers. This is usually successful because the size of the piece of meat these people have tried to swallow is truly astonishing: the *average* size found is as large as a pack of cigarettes; the largest piece found at autopsy was *7-1/4 inches long!* Apparently these people, because of ill-fitting or absent dentures, fall into the habit of swallowing larger and larger pieces of food. Finally, under the influence of alcohol in most cases, they tried to swallow a piece that was just a bit too large. Death occurred in minutes. In view of the fact that it has been estimated that almost 4,000 people a year die of this condition in the United States, it was felt that widely publicizing the existence of such a condition, along with its simple cure, would help prevent these deaths.

Recently, however, a new technique especially for smaller particles has been approved by the American Medical Association that might even be more effective than reaching into the back of a person's throat, since the latter method might not be successful in dislodging a morsel of food small enough to have actually begun to pass down the windpipe before getting stuck. The new method is called the Heimlich Maneuver after the doctor who first described it. It is based on the fact that just the way air cannot get into the lungs when the person tries to gasp, so air is not able to escape from the victim's lungs. Now, the normal lungs act as a bellows, being in a somewhat closed position when the person exhales. The principle of the Heimlich Maneuver is to so clasp the person in one's arms that one forces air out of the lungs. Since there is only one way for the air to escape and that is up and out through the windpipe, this forceful maneuver usually causes the expulsion not only of the trapped air but also of the offending morsel which is forcibly pushed out of the windpipe by the rush of air behind it. Standing behind the victim, wrap your arms around his waist. Grasp your fist with your other hand and place the thumb side of your fist against the abdomen, slightly above the navel and below the rib cage. Press your fist into the victim's abdomen with a *quick, upward* thrust. Repeat several times, if necessary. So successful has this maneuver become that it has been officially adopted by the American Medical Association, and it has been recommended that it be given wide publicity.

COLD WEATHER INJURIES

Chief among cold weather injuries would be injury due to the cold itself. A distinction may be made between exposure to damp cold when temperatures are around freezing and exposure to dry cold usually with temperatures below freezing. Such conditions as immersion foot (trench foot) and chilblains belong to the former category while true frostbite belongs to the latter.

The damp cold injuries have sometimes been called frostnips. The involved areas (usually the ears, nose, chin, or extremities rather than the more central areas of the body) are usually firm, white, and cold. If treated quickly the skin soon returns to normal; if not, sunburnlike damage such as peeling or blistering can occur in a few days, and the area may subsequently remain quite sensitive to cold. Immersion foot results in a clammy swelling often with superficial skin breakdown. This may often be associated with long-term symptoms such as cold susceptibility and generalized skin sensitivity. Frostbite itself causes the involved area to be cold, hard, white, and numb; rewarming causes the involved skin to be blotchy-red, swollen, and painful. If caught early enough, these symptoms may disappear, leaving few if any significant residual problems; however, if not treated early, true gangrene may result.

Currently, the time-honored methods of treating this condition by slowly rewarming the affected areas or by rubbing them with or without snow are now considered not good, and should be avoided. The suggestions for the relatively mild frostnip is to treat it by rapid rewarming of the affected part with a warm object or by body heat of the hands if they are not affected. Such rapid rewarmings are recommended for the more severe frostbite, with the best method being a warm bath, if it is available. Hot drinks to warm the body internally, heating pads, or even hot water bottles are considered effective. A word of caution is in order regarding the rewarming temperatures; they should be only slightly above the normal body temperature of 98.6°. A rewarming temperature of a 100° or so, such as one finds in a person with a low grade fever, is ideal. The temperature of whatever rewarming method is used must never exceed 110° Fahrenheit. That is why the suggestion to rewarm by using body heat of oneself or of a warm companion is so often made. When water is used for rewarming, the skin must be very thoroughly dried to avoid any further injury.

If the skin looks obviously damaged, a clean protective dressing is a good thing to use, and of course blisters should never be broken. One final word regarding treatment; when hot drinks are used, it is generally recommended that they have no alcohol content.

Of course the best thing to do about cold injuries is to avoid them. Warm multilayered clothing is always a good idea, and special protection for hands and feet should be provided; especially keep in mind the avoidance of tight wristbands and tight socks and shoes. Since 25 to 50% of body heat can be lost through the head, warm head gear is definitely needed. The things that can contribute to cold injuries, while obvious, are often ignored. They include fatigue, hunger, very young or very old age, chronic circulatory problems, high altitude, wind chill, alcohol, and fear.

Another winter health problem is the occurrence of an acute coronary attack, usually in a man, usually during or shortly after he has been doing some shoveling. I recall years ago, when I was in medical school, a professor saying with a perfectly straight face, that no man

over 45 should ever shovel snow again. While this may be good news
to those who are over 45 and lazy, it is not practical. Surely, anyone
over 45 who is completely "out of shape" in that he almost never
does any physical exertion probably should not be shoveling snow.
For the rest, common sense again rules the day: Work slowly; don't
try to scoop too much snow at any one time; if at all possible, break
up the job into two or three relatively brief sessions rather than the
one prolonged exhausting session. If possible, enlist younger members of the family to help. Finally, go inside in the presence of the
chest discomfort that in any way even begins to differ from the kind
of familiar muscular feeling one has when one has done some unusual exertion.

With loads of snow it is good advice also to avoid running into a
significant low back problem. A little low back muscle stiffness is one
thing, but an acute occurrence of disc pressure on a nerve can lay you
up in bed for weeks. While such symptoms can sometimes have a
dramatic, relatively immediate onset, more often the back problem
manifests itself a day or two later. In such cases, without current pain
to serve as a warning, the best advice is to follow the advice given
above for coronary avoidance, and add to it that if you have ever
truly had a medically diagnosed disc problem, you probably
shouldn't be shoveling snow at all.

Finally, always be careful when walking on icy patches. A momen-
tary lack of attention (of which I was guilty) can result in a seemingly
minor fall (which I had) which can lead to anything from a broken
wrist or ankle to a broken back (which latter I sustained) and months
of recrimination.

CYSTIC MASTITIS

The most common of all breast conditions is a benign one called
chronic cystic mastitis.

"Chronic cystic mastitis" or "cystic mastitis" as it is also called is,
in a way, a set of misnomers since generally the *itis* ending on a condition usually signifies an infectious or inflammatory condition
("tonsillitis," "appendicitis," etc.), while this condition is neither one
nor the other. Perhaps "cystic disease" would be a better name for it.

The hallmark of the condition is that there are cysts in the breasts, usually more than one cyst, often in both breasts. If there are *no* cysts, then we don't have "cystic mastitis." Such cysts do not have to be large. As a matter of fact, the condition probably begins with microscopically small cysts which cannot be felt. They probably start as localized swellings of the normal duct tissues of the breast which then go on to enlarge and become palpable by the patient.

So common is cystic disease of the breast that it has been estimated that one in every ten women will eventually develop it. It occurs generally in middle life (ages 35 to 50) though it has even occurred as isolated unilateral lesions in young women in their middle 20's. Generally the condition subsides and disappears with the menopause. It is extremely unusual for the condition to be found in women over 55.

Forty percent of those women with gross (or palpable) cystic disease subsequently develop new cysts at intervals of from less than 1 year up to 30 years after the initial cyst (which initially appears, in over 10% of women, in *both* breasts). New cysts are usually widely scattered throughout the breast tissue and not necessarily in contact with or even in the vicinity of the first cyst. After the age of 40, women with gross cystic disease tend to develop more and more cysts at shorter and shorter intervals. Thus the disease actually reaches its most active phase during the premenopausal years and disappears after the completion of the menopause.

That the condition does not develop until a considerable number of years after the full onset of complete female ovarian hormonal activity coupled with the fact that it disappears with the menopause suggests that it is, in some way, related to an abnormality of ovarian function. It is not known whether this is due to an excess of estrogen or to some other type of hormonal dysfunction.

Cystic disease of the breast often produces no symptoms; and usually the patient is unaware of the disease until she accidentally discovers it, as, for example, when she is doing her monthly breast self-examination. Some women may have painful cysts or they may be tender to palpation. The symptoms may either be present continuously or may appear only in the premenstrual phase of the menstrual cycle. The pain and tenderness are more apt to be present when the cyst has enlarged rapidly. This discomfort may be related to the tension of the fluid within the cyst since aspiration of the cyst fluid almost invariably gives relief.

A peculiarity of these cysts is that they develop quickly, often before the menstrual period, and may diminish in size just as rapidly (usually after the period is over). One good clue to a condition being cystic disease and not breast cancer is that when a competent observer definitely observes a shrinkage in the size of the swelling, it is usually cystic disease. Finally, discharge from the nipple occurs rarely, if at all, in cystic disease.

Cysts of the breast are usually round and well-outlined from normal tissue. Of course, they are always fluid-filled; and the amount of fluid contained determines the consistency of the cyst. Soft cysts normally mean little fluid under low pressure while firm cysts usually are like that because they are tightly distended with fluid. Long-standing cysts may become thickened by fibrous tissue and this would, in turn, tend to contribute to their firmness. Unlike cancers, cysts are usually relatively moveable in the surrounding breast tissue. Some cysts which are close to the surface of the skin are often called "blue-domed" cysts because of their rounded, bluish appearance.

The diagnosis of cystic disease of the breast usually turns out to be the treatment for it also. The way to establish the nature of the condition is aspiration of the cyst. This does *not* mean that every breast lump should be aspirated but if the lump occurs in a woman of the right age (between 30 and 55), if the growth feels like a cyst (rounded, well-outlined, and moveable), if it is not hard and is not associated with a pulling of the skin down toward it, then it may very well be aspirated. Of course, if the patient has already had previously proved cystic disease of the breast, this would help toward a similar diagnosis once again.

One peculiarity of these cysts is that for an unknown reason once the fluid is removed it almost never reaccumulates. If aspiration does not yield fluid, then the patient should be hospitalized for a biopsy of the lesion. Sometimes, at surgery, it will turn out to be a cyst after all but one with not too much fluid and lots of thickened fibrous tissue around it.

One final sober note: While cystic mastitis is not a cancer, women who have this condition are four times as likely to develop breast cancer as women in the general population. So, even though it *was* cystic disease, a woman should not neglect breast self-examination monthly or regular checkups by her physician.

FAD DISEASES

Just like so many other items of popular American culture, medicine, too, has its fads. To call them "nondiseases" might be a little too harsh; but certainly the fad conditions, if they exist at all, are never very serious. Some people seem to need to have a label of illness pinned upon them, though there are very few people who wish to have that label be of a serious illness. There aren't too many people lining up to be told that they have cancer. As a matter of fact, many an unfortunate patient who does indeed have cancer is most reluctant to talk about it and often will try to keep it secret. Not so with fad diseases. They are worn as a "badges of honor," and the lucky recipient often seems to find every opportunity to let the world know of his restrictive affliction. It is almost as if the presence of the fad disease serves as some kind of peculiar status symbol. The truth may be that people who have fad diseases may, indeed, be less than well; but it may very well be that their problem doesn't lie in the physical area.

In the 1920's and 1930's, colitis was the disease to have. Just about all of us have some bowel changes during certain times of our lives: brief periods of change in pattern and other periods of stomach awareness such as cramping. Actually, most of us would deny such symptoms, and only if carefully pressed, will everyone eventually realize that indeed they have had such symptoms occasionally. For a significant group of patients, however, these symptoms proved to be disturbing enough for them to consult their physicians and, before we knew it, a popular disease was born. From a search of the historical medical records, it is quite evident that the very serious condition, ulcerative colitis, was not at all what they were talking about. Nor does it seem that they were talking about the much less serious, but not much more common condition, spastic or mucous colitis; although there does seem to have been some overlap between the fad colitis and the mildest forms of spastic colitis.

In the 50's and 60's and, it seems, perhaps forever, we saw the birth of allergies. Allergies were used to explain everything from nasal mucus to rectal mucus. Headaches, chest tightness, stomach cramps, skin rashes, itchiness with rashes, peculiar behavior, you name it—allergy caused it. The prompt recital by the faddist of those things which he must avoid on the pain of death dulled, even further, many a dragging cocktail party. Visits to allergists became a social routine, and one can still hear people outvying each other: "You're lucky, you're only allergic to 14 things; I'm allergic to 27." This is not to say that there are not a few people, a very few people, who are really and seriously allergic to some items. The person who gets hives or choking sensations from penicillin may die from a future exposure, and this may very well be the most serious of allergies. Some people will get rashes from strawberries, or chocolate, or fish. Even hives can result. For such people, reexposure to the offending item will cause a recurrence of the rash or hives; but, quite obviously, neither of these conditions poses much of a fatal threat to the patient. Some people will have an internal respiratory manifestation from the allergen in the way of shortness of breath or constriction of the throat. While more serious than the skin manifestations, nonetheless, such exposures rarely prove overwhelming. All of these, however, are the people who are truly allergic; and they are indeed a very small number. Meanwhile, we have these other patients marching through life and into their doctors' offices waving high their banners of "I am allergic."

And now, another fad is born: hypoglycemia. This has an especially great appeal because, to begin with, it is barely pronounceable; and one is absolutely assured of almost everyone in one's audience being totally unaware of what you are talking about. When the patient is finished with an explanation of what the disease is, he sounds so bright and scientifically "with it" that one suspects he may have a connection with the medical profession after all but is too modest to tell us about it. A casting down of the eyes and fleeting smile at the corner of one's lips is especially helpful in conveying that impression before one looks up earnestly into the face of one's captive audience and regales them with the specific details of one's own hypoglycemic episodes.

True hypoglycemia is very, very rare. The most common cause is due to excessive amounts of insulin such as is caused by a tumor of the pancreas. Sometimes diabetics (diabetes is a disease of hyperglycemia) also will experience a hypoglycemia. There are a few congenital abnormalities of enzymes of the body's metabolism which can cause this condition also. All of these are rare. All of these are serious, and nobody in his right mind would like to have any of them and, as a matter of fact, they don't. The fad hypoglycemia is something whose cause is totally mysterious and which afflicts the nervous patient not only systemically but also in his tongue for he can scarcely keep the latter from wagging and telling people all about his symptoms, one of the sure signs of a fad disease.

For those poor unfortunate nonhypoglycemics among our readers, a brief definition is in order: Hypoglycemia means low blood sugar. The normal fasting blood sugar in adults should be between 70 and 110 milligrams percent. The confusion that has made hypoglycemics of people and physicians wealthier is the placing of too much emphasis on what are the rigid boundaries of normal. The reasoning goes something like this—if 70 milligrams of blood sugar is the lower limit of normal, there must be something dreadfully wrong with a blood sugar of 55 or 60. Unfortunately, the 70 to 110 figure is a universal mean clustering, so to speak; and it is not at all unusual to find a number of people with blood sugar significantly lower than 70 without any abnormalities afflicting these people whatsoever. If, however, the person goes to a doctor with vague symptoms ranging from headache, tingling of the fingers, nausea, trembling, spots in front of the eyes to generalized nervousness, and the doctor happens to find a blood sugar of 55, *voilà*—a new disease is born. The patient has a label, and the doctor has some way of explaining what he had no idea of beforehand.

Specialists in metabolic diseases insist that in order to have a true diagnosis of hypoglycemia, the blood sugar must be below 40 milligrams percent. If that rigid criteria were to be applied to the current host of hypoglycemics, they would evaporate and, like the fabled Arabs, "silently steal away."

HICCUPS

We all have them sometimes and we are all experts in getting rid of them, but every once in a while our favorite technique doesn't work and we slip from impatience to annoyance, to discomfort, and sometimes panic, especially in those rare cases where they can last for hours. What we are talking about is singultus, more commonly known as hiccups.

Hiccuping is an involuntary spasm of the muscles of inspiration, usually of the chief muscle of inspiration, the diaphragm, followed by an abrupt closure of the top of the windpipe which causes the characteristic sound. There probably is no one in the world who has not experienced a hiccup, especially after eating or drinking. Some people get them after prolonged throat clearing; but in some rare instances, hiccuping may be a symptom of disease.

Let us briefly deal with the serious conditions since they are rare and generally do not respond to the home remedies or even the more medically acceptable ones that will be discussed towards the end of the article. One of the longest nerves in the body is the vagus nerve, which comes from the brain and is responsible for much of the involuntary nervous system-muscle activity of the internal organs of the chest and abdomen, reaching down as far as into the intestine. Anything which irritates the vagus nerve can trigger hiccuping, and among the serious causes of the condition are certain cases of gastritis, peritonitis, pleurisy, and inflammation around the sac of the heart, which is called pericarditis. Even more rare, but perhaps most troublesome of all is central hiccuping, by which we mean that the cause is not due to some irritation or affliction of the vagus nerve or its innervated structures of the body itself but rather due to an irritative focus in a certain part of the brain which then centrally triggers the vagus nerve to cause contraction of the diaphragm to cause hiccuping. One serious medical condition, uremia, which is the final stage of long-standing, generally untreated or untreatable kidney disease, is also often associated with very troublesome hiccuping whose origin is now believed to be of central origin as described above.

At times when no cause can be found for the hiccuping, psychological tension factors have been blamed for it; but the current medical thinking is that there really is no evidence to support this indictment of the psyche in causing the symptom. Chronic alcoholism has also been blamed as a cause of hiccups, and whether this is from a nerve irritation or a gastritis associated with alcohol has never been decided. Most of us, however, who have hiccups usually find that they occur after something that has temporarily irritated the involved structures, such as swallowing hot or irritating substances.

Perhaps no realm of medical symptomatology is as much open to mumbo-jumbo remedies as is hiccuping. The funny thing is that many of these mumbo-jumbo remedies work, which is partly the reason the psychogenic origin of hiccuping has been given some prominence over the years.

Before going into detail about the various remedies, however, be assured that in many cases hiccups just stop by themselves. I will try to cover as many of Grandma's home remedies, as well as the currently accepted medical measures, as possible.

One medical text attributes success to the following measures merely because they serve to divert the patient's attention. Those of us who swear by them as an effective cure for hiccups know that such a text doesn't know what it is talking about. One of the great cures is to scare a person by coming up behind him and shouting. When one adds a slap on the back to a shout, indeed one has a dramatic cure, if the patient doesn't die of fright in the process. Painful stimuli of various sorts have also been recommended to distract one's self from hiccuping. I personally don't recommend them since pinching and squeezing one's self can often be a heck of a lot worse than just the hiccups. The most famous of all remedies for hiccups is probably taking a deep breath and holding it, and holding it, and holding it, until your eyes feel as if they are popping out of your head, your face looks like a cousin to the beet, and you feel you are going to die from lack of oxygen any second now. The really operative factor in breath holding is the accumulation of carbon dioxide in the blood and lungs which somehow serves to stop the hiccups. As a consequence, some people have learned to slip paper bags over their heads if they can't stop hiccuping because, in a paper bag, you are rebreathing your own expired air which contains, obviously, much more carbon dioxide than the normal inhaled air. This results in an increased volume of carbon dioxide in the blood and lungs and, *violà,* no more hiccups. For those devotees of the paper bag, one should remind them that plastic bags are not be used since they can occlude the nostrils as well as set a very dangerous example to children. My own personal never-fail remedy is to swallow six sips of water, count aloud one, two, three, etc., after each sip, making sure no hiccups intervene in the counting sequence. If they do, you have to start all over again. Others find that sipping ice water will break the cycle. Still others try regular deep breathing. One medical text advises inhaling strong fumes, but I consider that in the same category as painful stimuli, one where the cure is almost worse than the disease.

Among many other not-so-famous remedies of Grandma's is inducing vomiting. Also in this category, it is recommended that one pull out the tongue vigorously (not out of the head completely but just pulling it forward from the lips). Also highly recommended is swallowing dry bread. Pressure on the eyeballs is also listed in one of my medical texts (again don't press on both eyeballs at once because you can drop dead if you do). Others feel that the application of various remedies over the belly is in order and recommend mustard plasters, ice packs, or even spraying ethyl chloride over the skin of the stomach area.

The *New England Journal of Medicine* once ran a series of letters regarding cures which included swallowing a teaspoonful of sugar or (and again I put this in the "cure worse than the disease" category) drinking a small amount of vinegar. One of my medical texts recommends washing out the stomach, "galvanic stimulation of the phrenic nerve" (unfortunately I know what it means but I wouldn't dare tell you). It also lists dilating the esophagus with a metal tube. The following is a direct quote from another medical text. "A simple method almost universally successful is to introduce a plastic or rubber suction catheter through the nose to a distance of 3 or 4 in., to stimulate the pharynx by a jerky to-and-fro movement. The method is suitable whether the cause is cerebral, thoracic, or abdominal, and can be used in either conscious or anesthetized patients. The sensitive area of stimulation is the midpharynx behind the uvula and opposite the second cervical vertebra." (This, as far as I am concerned, is a cure worse than death itself.) Since I have run out of space and my grandmother has just hung up on the telephone, this article will draw to a close. There are indeed a number of classy medical remedies involving chemicals with long names; but thank heavens, there is no room to go into that now.

HOARSENESS

One of the most frequent of all medical complaints is hoarseness. In the overwhelming majority of instances, it is of brief duration and is caused by a recent or current upper respiratory infection. There are, however, enough cases due to other causes that it might be worth reviewing some of the more common of these.

Hoarseness is *not* a vague sore throat; it has a specific meaning: Something has gone wrong, not in the throat, but rather lower down, in the voice box (or larynx, as it is called medically). What *has* gone wrong is that the vocal cords are no longer aligning perfectly when they vibrate to make sound.

The first matter to be settled in trying to figure out the cause of hoarseness is how long it has been present. If it has come on during the past week, one should then try to relate it to the presence of other symptoms. If there has recently been sneezing, nasal congestion, increased mucus production, postnasal drip, a feeling of blocking in the ears, some burning in the back of the throat, a cough, and maybe even a low-grade fever, the diagnosis of upper respiratory infection is obvious. A cold doesn't have to have all of these symptoms, but two or three of them recently present are enough to put any associated hoarseness in the "nothing-much-to-worry-about" category. Voice rest, plenty of liquids, and maybe some steam inhalations should clear up the symptoms in a few days. Many throat specialists also advise avoidance of smoking and hot spicy foods. They also feel that whispering is no real alternative since this strains the vocal cords as much as talking.

When there is recent onset of hoarseness in the absence of the symptoms of a cold, one should look toward unusual and excessive use of the voice or exposure to some irritant as the cause. An unusual vocal strain such as abnormally long periods of talking or yelling at a sports event may be responsible. Among the irritants that could be a factor in recent-onset hoarseness are smoking, backyard leaf and trash burning, and even at times heavy smog. The same recommendations as for hoarseness due to a cold should help to rapidly clear up the condition.

Then we move into the area of hoarseness of longer duration: weeks or months. Nowadays, the first thing that has to be considered is a history of heavy smoking or something like long-term exposure to noxious fumes. Heavy drinkers often develop a chronic, noninfectious hoarseness. Whether it's because they, at the same time, smoke too much or whether the actual heavy intake of alcohol is a factor is not clear. Irritant-type laryngitis often is most prominent in the morning; vocal-abuse hoarseness often tends to be worse toward the end of the day. Some systemic conditions that can be associated with hoarseness include marked underactivity of the thyroid glands. Diagnostic tests will reveal the condition, and replacement treatment with thyroid hormone should lead to a permanent cure. Even "the pill" is sometimes associated with hoarseness. In such cases, the hoarseness is usually mild and intermittent and is harmless. In most such cases your doctor will perform direct laryngoscopy to help rule out the more serious causes of hoarseness. This involves looking at the voice box with one of those doctor mirrors on the end of a long thin handle that one sees in the movies and TV doctor programs. If he has ruled out serious conditions, a conservative line of approach is indicated, consisting of absolute cessation of smoking, voice rest (at times extending to complete silence during specified periods of the day), and, again, plain old steam inhalations.

When the hoarseness is of long duration and is associated with a chronic cough, this probably indicates an active infection which must be treated. Hoarseness may be the first symptom of a tuberculosis that the patient has no idea he has. He may have been ignoring the fatigue, the weight loss, and the coughing, and the fever. However, the presence of hoarseness may bring him to the doctor for fear that it might be a sign of cancer.

While hoarseness associated with the coughing up of blood-streaked sputum may be due to a chronic irritation, it is often a signal of a deeper respiratory infection of the lungs. Such an infection can be bacterial (such as tuberculosis) or it can be caused by a fungus.

Now we come to the potentially even more serious causes of hoarseness: the various growths (including cancer) that can cause hoarseness. Two characteristics stand above all others in pointing the way to cancer of the larynx. They are *persistent* hoarseness and *constant* hoarseness. Usually such a hoarseness develops suddenly and very quickly after the start of the tumor growth, and it gets progressively worse in a short time. Attacks of hoarseness that clear up completely and then recur usually are not due to cancer since cancer-caused hoarseness is generally constant.

It is imperative for your doctor to examine your voice box when you have persistent, constant hoarseness of long duration. People expect that they should have pain of some sort with a cancer. However, pain and coughing are not ordinarily symptoms of an early stage of cancer of the vocal cords themselves, although sometimes pain can be a sign of voice box cancer that may eventually spread to the vocal cords, thus causing hoarseness.

Some of the doom and gloom associated with the word *growth* may be dispelled by the realization that not all growths are cancer. As a matter of fact, most lesions of the larynx will turn out not to be malignant. Among the nonmalignant voice box growths are leukoplakia, keratoses, polyps, and nodules. The former two are raised, localized thickenings of the vocal cords, while the latter two are actual projecting small lumps of growth tissue. All of these should be watched until they go away by themselves; if they don't, they should be removed for it is possible that a cancer can eventually develop in them.

Some of the rarer causes of hoarseness (by various different mechanisms) include rheumatoid arthritis, various neurological conditions which cause paralysis of the nerves controlling the vocal cords, and even certain cardiovascular conditions such as abnormal enlargements of the aorta.

But remember, the overwhelming majority of instances of hoarseness are of brief duration and are due to the common cold.

HYSTERECTOMY

The popular press has, from time to time, had some disturbing "exposés" of various medical practices including such accusations as that the American people are being subjected to fragmented medicine because of the large number of super-specialists being turned out by the American medical establishment. Not only has the family doctor, who took care of the entire person along with his wife and his children, almost completely vanished, but even the general internist who used to be available for almost total patient care is now supplanted, according to the claims, by the heart specialist, and the kidney specialist, and the liver specialist, and the lung specialist, and the blood specialist, and so on. We've even been told there are more neurosurgeons in the United States than in the rest of the world put together, with the unspoken but implied corollary that we either have much greater need for brain surgery in the United States than the rest of the world or we're going to get more brain surgery than the rest of the world even if we don't need it. Furthermore, statistics have been published that claim that Americans are subjected to scandalously large numbers of unnecessary operations with gallbladder removals and removals of the uterus leading the list.

In 1973, 690,000 hysterectomies were performed in the United States: that is, over six operations for every 1,000 women in America

—a higher rate than for any other major operation and one which if continued in the future would result in loss of the uterus by more than half the female population by the age of 65 years. There are some generally accepted reasons for performing hysterectomies with which very few physicians would argue. Among these are the presence of early, localized stages of potentially invasive cancers of the cervix or the body of the uterus itself. Much of the success in prolonging life in cancer patients is due to the prompt discovery of such very early malignancies with their subsequent removal. More controversial, however, would be the removal of the uterus for the discovery, for example, of a premalignant state on a Pap smear. Since such abnormal cells generally take months at least to become true malignancies, a number of physicians advise more frequent Pap tests to see if such premalignant cells were merely a false alarm, will remain as a premalignant condition, or will become an early case of "the real thing." Naturally, in the latter case, surgery would be in order; but since the progression from premalignant to malignant is by no means inevitable, there is much to be said for the camp that recommends watchful waiting rather than immediate surgery.

Fibroids are benign tumors of the uterus. They may hang freely by a narrow stalk in the cavity of the uterus; some of them are completely enclosed within the walls of the uterine muscle itself; while others may bulge outward from the external aspect of the womb into the surrounding peritoneal cavity. It is generally accepted that these tumors are completely responsive to hormones and their changing levels. As a result, it is almost universally true that once a woman has entered into her menopause, fibroids will shrink markedly or disappear altogether. Nonetheless, the question of the performance of a hysterectomy because of the presence of fibroids is still actively debated among gynecologists. Some would advocate removal of the uterus if the fibroids (especially those which project outward into the peritoneal cavity) are causing symptoms by pressing on adjacent pelvic structures. Others feel that such pressure phenomena are more of an inconvenience than a serious medical problem and would suggest waiting until after the menopause to see the extent, if any, of the symptoms, therefore deferring surgery. On the other hand, fibroids can bleed, especially those which protrude into the cavity of the uterus. If repeated episodes of bleeding are not brought under control by scrapings, most surgeons would then recommend hysterectomy for the condition even though fibroids are not malignant. As a matter of fact, most surgeons would recommend hysterectomy for repeated episodes of uterine bleeding which are not responsive to hormonal therapy regardless of the cause.

A more controversial reason for the removal of the uterus is for surgery being performed for diseases in the adjacent structures. For example, if one is going to operate upon and remove chronic disease in the ovarian and fallopian tube area, a number of surgeons would advocate the removal of the uterus at the same time. This would be especially the case if the disease in the adjacent areas is a malignancy, to reduce the likelihood of spread to the uterus. Of course, if the patient desires to retain the possibility of future pregnancies, adjacent area disease can be removed without a hysterectomy.

If the ligaments which support the uterus in the lower part of the body have become weakened or stretched due to disease, there is a tendency for the uterus to descend lower than it should and even to prolapse (protrude). Unless there is a very good reason not to, in these cases many doctors would agree that a hysterectomy should be performed. Sometimes hysterectomy is necessary for a catastrophic complication of pregnancy, and for this there would be very few, if any, arguments among surgeons. However, the performance of a hysterectomy as a means of birth control (for example, if performed at the time of a therapeutic abortion for an unwanted pregnancy) is indeed a bone of real contention among gynecologists. One gyencologist stated that if a woman is 35 or 40 years old and has an organ that is disease-prone and of little or no further use, it might as well be removed.

It certainly is true that medicine is unaware of any necessary function of the uterus except for the sheltering and nourishment of the unborn fetus. So far as is known, the uterus does not secrete any hormones or other necessary chemicals for the maintenance of the body's internal metabolism. Nonetheless, some of the dissenters feel strongly that prophylactic removal of the uterus not only would result in a lot of unnecessary surgery, but also would have some significant nongynecological complications. Psychiatrists, as well as some gynecologists, have stated that even though the chief function of the uterus may no longer be operative, there is much to be said for its retention if only from the point of view of the patient's total self-image as a woman. They have pointed out that loss of bodily parts or functions is frequently accompanied by some degree of depression, and one study showed that fully 1/3 of patients who had had a hysterectomy within the preceding 3 years suffered from depression and required antidepressant drugs—which figure was five times greater than the occurrence of depression in patients of similar ages who had not had the surgery. A refinement of this dramatic study has led to the conclusion that there may be certain categories of patients who are more likely than others to experience depression after a hysterectomy: those who have experienced prior emotional disturbances, women with marital disturbances, women without pelvic disease, and younger women, especially if they are under the age of 40.

There has been recent publicity given to the idea of second opinions for nonemergency surgery. Some Blue Cross-Blue Shield plans have even instituted payments for such opinions. Since hysterectomy almost always falls into that category, it would be an excellent idea for all patients to whom the operation is recommended to get such a second opinion. Unnecessary surgery would thus be avoided, while necessary surgery would not be forestalled.

LYMPH NODES

Having been warned to be wary of the appearance of any suspicious lump in the body, many persons will go the doctor because of some of these swellings only to be told, "That's just an enlarged lymph node." Unfortunately, the doctor, assuming that everybody knows what that means, doesn't elaborate further; and the patient often seems reassured but, if anything, is even more mystified.

Lymph-node enlargement is very common not only because it is secondary to one of man's most common ills, infection, but also because there are so many lymph nodes in the body. It has been estimated that 500 to 600 lymph nodes are scattered throughout the body, some being no larger than the head of a pin and others normally being up to 1/2 to 3/4 of an inch in size. They can be located almost anywhere in the body, both superficially, near the skin and deep within the body itself. The chief areas where lymph nodes cluster and thus are more easily felt are: on the inside part of the upper elbow area, in the armpits, in the junction between the thigh and the lower abdomen, and in the neck. In the neck they are found not only under the jaw bone and down along either side of the neck, but they can also be found behind the ear. These are the only ones that can really be felt on physical examination because the deeper ones, such as those around the aorta and the large blood vessels, are much too deep to be felt even when they are enlarged.

The lymph nodes are way stations, so to speak, of a sort of secondary circulatory system which parallels the main system. Our main circulatory system consists of blood leaving the heart through the arteries, then going to all parts of the body and returning via the veins to the heart for recirculation. The chief purpose of the primary circulatory system is to supply the body with oxygen and essential nutrients from our food. The lymph system originates in the tissues and is really the great sewer system of the body. Debris from the breakdown of cells, bacteria, and other infectious organisms and foreign particles that have gotten into the body are among the chief products that are filtered out of the body via the lymph system.

The lymph flow is away from the tissue site converging towards the clearance centers or lymph nodes and eventually dumping into the veins. The lymph nodes themselves, besides being way stations in the convergence of the lymph channels, also have two other important functions. The first is to act as mechanical filters against all foreign material mentioned above and the second is to be very active in combatting all the various infectious conditions that afflict us.

The lymph glands are packed with lymphocytes, which are those cells in our body which not only make antibodies against foreign proteins (the B-type lymphocyte), but also can become active themselves in migrating throughout the system and helping to ingest and destroy the invading germs (the T-type of lymphocyte).

In a normal person, even on physical examination, very few, if any, lymph nodes can be felt. When lymph nodes enlarge rapidly, such as when we have an infection anatomically near that lymph node and its cluster, the patient will notice a tenderness to touch and sometimes even pain associated with swelling. When the lymph nodes enlarges slowly, as in Hodgkin's disease and other types of cancerous conditions that can afflict the lymph nodes, both tenderness and pain are often absent, and the patient notices the swelling primarily. When a lymph node is associated with infection or a relatively benign condition, it is not firm, not hard, it is moveable, not adherent to the underlying structures, and usually it is single rather than part of a matted-together chain of lymph nodes.

When there is redness over an enlarged node along with tenderness, then it is almost certainly due to an internal infection, be it bacterial or, on occasion, even viral or caused by a fungus. Swellings of the lymph nodes due to various malignancies are usually not associated with overlying skin redness.

Lymph nodes can enlarge either locally or in a widespread fashion. Local enlargement usually is associated with a nearby focus of infection which drains into the lymph node, although Hodgkin's disease is notorious in that it too usually begins as a local lymph node swelling. Generalized enlargement of all or most of the lymph nodes usually is a much more serious condition, however; it reflects an infection which has gotten out of hand because it cannot be controlled by itself in the local lymph nodes and is thus spreading throughout the body, or it may represent a primary disease of the lymph nodes (such as some types of lymphomas or leukemias).

There are some quite specific areas of lymph node enlargement: Enlargement of the lymph nodes behind and below the ear almost always means German measles. In the old days, head lice used to also cause a similar swelling. Infectious mononucleosis, which has now finally been attributed to a virus infection, characteristically causes enlargement of the lymph nodes in the neck, although other lymph nodes may also be enlarged. Infections of the foot almost always cause enlargement of the lymph nodes in the groin.

Though seen much less often because the conditions are less prevalent and the treatment is more successful, there were certain chronic infections as well as acute infections that could cause lymph node enlargement. Chief among these were syphilis and tuberculosis. The syphilitic lymph nodes are usually a local enlargement, draining the focus of primary infection. The tuberculous lymph nodes are usually more generalized and often appear in the neck (scrofula). Tuberculosis also tends to cause the enlargement of the internal lymph nodes which are not usually felt on examination.

Some of the rare causes of lymph node enlargement are the taking of certain drugs to control epilepsy, Addison's disease, and overactive thyroid.

It should be evident from all this that the discovery of an enlarged lymph node requires a thorough examination of the patient to determine the cause. For example, while cervical lymph gland enlargement could be caused by something as minor as a gum infection, it might be due to a dental abscess or strep throat, or, more rarely, Hodgkin's disease, infectious mononuculeosis or tuberculosis. Besides a complete physical examination, blood tests may often be necessary to determine not only if an infection is present but also what type of infection is present. Sometimes, skin tests are indicated to help determine the cause. It should be emphasized that in most cases lymph node enlargement is a reflection of disease elsewhere and, as such, treatment should not be directed necessarily solely towards the lymph node enlargement. Rather, the primary cause should be elucidated and treated and in the great majority of cases, the lymph node enlargement will subside and take care of itself within 2 to 4 weeks if the inciting cause has been removed.

CHRISTMAS OVERINDULGENCE

It is probably medically true that if the only time we overindulged in food and drink were during such an annual holiday as Christmas, there would be no detriment to our health. Unfortunately, in spite of today's inflation and predicted recession with their attendant economic uncertainties, the majority of us still live in one of the most affluent countries in the history of civilization. As a consequence, for far too many Americans, the once-a-year orgy-feast has become a relatively frequent occurrence: Christmas, New Year's, "that special birthday," Thanksgiving, "that special anniversary," when you're feeling low, when you're feeling high, and so on. Now, *that* gravy train does lead to the medical diseases of overindulgence.

Before examining some of the consequences, we might consider one incident that can happen even to the "once-a-year" binger. This true episode was reported in the *New England Journal of Medicine* a few years ago. While it didn't occur during the Christmas season, nonetheless it did involve the kind of gorging that does occur at this time of year, and it serves our purpose well because the patient died as a result of his overindulgence.

This case involved a young sportsman of college age who, in an attempt to bring his weight under control and actually bring about a significant weight reduction, went on a very rigid diet devoted almost exclusively to protein intake with minimal quantities of fattening carbohydrates and fats. He continued this diet for weeks, successfully achieving his goal of weight reduction. When the competitive sports event for which he had been getting in condition was over, he indulged in a 1-day orgy of eating that resulted in the probable ingestion of between 4,000 and 6,000 calories, many of which were of fats and the carbohydrate classification known as sweets. He was dead the next day.

Autopsy revealed in essence a form of pancreatic apoplexy. In retrospect, what must have happened was that this young man, in following his rigid diet for a prolonged period of time, had put his pancreas "to sleep." The need for it to put out its normal (or, in the case of an obese person, its above normal) quota of digestive enzymes was markedly diminished. Not being called upon for such major functioning, the pancreas was, so to speak, stunned by the avalanche of calories that hit it on that 1 fatal day. The pancreas, having been virtually shut down, tried to gear up in 1 day for full production and it couldn't do it. One may consider that it choked to death and burst in the attempt. So, even the rare orgy can do the trick for us under the right circumstances.

Chronic overindulgence in food and drink usually doesn't result in instant death, but rather leads to the slow accumulation of bodily derangements responsible for the national epidemic of cardiovascular disease we are experiencing here in the United States. Every known statistical study has implicated diabetes as a significant factor in cardiovascular disease which, in turn, is the nation's #1 killer. Certainly there is a minority of young, thin diabetics who develop this unfortunate disease early in life as a result of genetic predisposition. The great majority of diabetics, however, are fat, middle-aged people. If they ate less, especially of the rich foods, and brought their weight down to what is an ideal weight for them, their disease would either be more easily controlled or might actually slide back into nonexistence for 1, 2, 3, or more years.

Rare indeed is the thin, young person who has a high cholesterol count. Such an unfortunate person usually has this condition on a genetic basis and will indeed suffer the cardiovascular consequences of the abnormal elevation in his blood fats. On the other hand, the majority of people with "hyperblood fats" eat and drink far too well—no, strike that out—far too badly. They are no strangers to hefty portions of beef two, three, or even more times a week. What would a meal be without a nice, rich dessert with lots of whipped cream or, if that's too fattening, "just one scoop of ice cream: well, all right, make it a small one-and-a-half scoops." Sure, a few drinks before a meal and one or two during a meal may help raise their triglycerides, but it also helps raise their digestive juices, their sense of camaraderie, and their spirit of enjoyment. And what is a good dinner without them?

Medical studies have shown repeatedly that these big orgiastic jolts of calories are very bad for the body's economy and control of fats and sugars, over and above the fact that such chronic overindulgence leads to obesity.

Let us turn our gaze now towards alcohol, that soother of jangled nerves, that boon to bosom friendship, that duller of sense and sensations, that energizer of the highway killer instinct. We all know that chronic drunkenness is a "no-no," but "surely alcohol has nothing to do with heart disease." Guess again! An unknown but very significant percentage of hypertensives don't have anything wrong with their body's anatomy or chemical makeup. The only thing underlying their hypertension is chronic overindulgence in alcohol. In those for whom the fog lifts and they finally see the light, their blood pressure invariably and inevitably comes down to normal and stays there. Dr. Jeremiah Stamler, one of America's leading heart specialists, has said that in his opinion alcohol is the chief culprit in the elevated triglyceride blood fats that so many Americans are afflicted with. So, besides the fact that it can eat a hole in your stomach, raise your blood pressure, increase your triglyceride count, kill you, and make you drive so that you kill others, alcohol also lowers your body's natural resistance to infection.

These overindulgences are the diseases that result from factors over which we *do have control. We* decide what to eat and what to drink, and how much. We do indeed have the potential of being, and may very well already be, the intellectual and social acme of life here on earth. But is the behavior which we call overindulgence consonant with the kind of maturity and wisdom that should come along with such a position? Speaking for myself if not for all my colleagues in the medical profession, I must say that we are discouraged by having to treat people whose diseases could have been prevented by the simple avoidance of bad habits—eating and otherwise. My advice would be to try to get *more* by using, consuming—yes, eating and drinking—

less. Underdo it, rather than *overdo* it. In other words, "cool" it when you "Yule" it. That way, I suggest, you'll have a much merrier Christmas.

ROCK AND ROLL NOISE POLLUTION

When one hears about pollution of the environment nowadays, the first thoughts that come to mind are about chemicals in the water and soil and chemicals in the air. Well, if we accept the definition of pollution as being any environmental contaminant that can cause damage, of any kind, to various forms of plant or animal life, then we may be overlooking one of the most damaging of all pollutants if we fail to keep in mind the damage caused by noise—in this case I mean noise of a very specific kind—rock and roll music.

Let me hasten to add that I personally believe that some of the best music available today is rock and roll music so this article should in no way be considered as an indictment of that music as a form—but it is an indictment of the extreme volume of loudness at which so much of rock and roll is performed. One of the main articles in an issue of the *New England Journal of Medicine* was entitled, "Auditory Fatigue and Permanent Hearing Defects from Rock-and-Roll Music," and its findings were startling.

The study was a scientific analysis of just how much dangerous noise was being put into the environment of devout "rockers." Thus, they found that at a local discotheque (in Connecticut, where the study was conducted), a typical reading on a sound-level meter was 110 db at a distance of 30 feet from the loudspeaker! To give some idea of what this means in comparative terms, here's a list of some common sounds and their db ratings:

Whispering	30 db
Normal conversation	60 db
Bedside table clock	75 db
Normal traffic sounds	80 db
Sound of garbage collection	85 db
Trumpet player	90 db
Street pneumatic hammers	95 db
Jet plane take-off	135 db

Generally, whenever one goes to the 90-db or above range, one begins to be concerned about damage to hearing.

With that background, one can see that 110 db, 30 feet away from the loudspeakers, is really loud. Undoubtedly it was even louder when closer to the loudspeakers. What conclusions were drawn from all this? There is at first a temporary shift downward in acuteness of hearing which then needs longer and longer periods for full recovery to ensue. There is a point, however, at which the researchers felt that permanent loss would result. They concluded that 2 hours at 110 db (and certainly it isn't unusual for people to spend 2 hours at a discotheque) would leave an "unusually severe" downward shift in hearing thresholds in about 14% of young men affected. They suggested that in order to cut down that damage to only 2% affected, the db level would have to be reduced to about 100 db.

Their final conclusion is startling: "It is not likely that society could insist that our young restrict themselves to so mild a sound as 100 db for 2 hours, so we shall have to reconcile ourselves to damaging the 14% most susceptible and later providing a variety of social rehabilitative and Medicare support to which these persons certainly will eventually turn."

End of article. What shall we do about it? When one considers how exercised and worried people are about air pollution due to dust, dirt, or smog (which certainly has *not* been proved to cause anywhere near 14% damage in persons exposed) or water pollution from various detergent solutions and wastes (which have been shown to damage fish life but *have yet to be shown to have caused any damage to humans*), then it is surprising how lackadaisical we are about something which has been *proved* to damage 14% of those exposed.

Do away with rock and roll? Of course not! Lower its volume? Why not?

SMOKING

There is now no real honest medical doubt that prolonged exposure (15–20 years or more) to large amounts of tobacco smoke (over one pack of inhaled cigarettes per day) has a direct causative relation to lung cancer. There is one ray of light in the lung cancer picture: It has been indisputably proven that it's never too late to stop. If one can get by the first 6 to 12 months after stopping cigarettes without developing lung cancer, then the likelihood of developing it subsequent to that period of time is almost as remote as if one had never smoked in the first place! Cigarette smokers have at least a ten times greater chance of developing lung cancer than nonsmokers; ex-smokers have *less than* twice as much chance as nonsmokers.

While the chances of developing lung cancer diminish with the cessation of cigarette smoking, the damage that has been done to the lungs during years of inhaling cigarette smoke is irreversible. Cigarette smoke irritates and inflames the bronchi leading from the windpipe to the lungs. The results are chronic bronchitis with cough and phlegm and emphysema with its attendant shortness of breath and often permanent disability. Yet even here there's a bright side: Lung scarring and ruptured air sacs don't return to normal, but much of the current inflammation can subside once cigarette smoking is stopped. I've had many patients tell me that their daily morning cough and phlegm stopped completely within weeks of going off cigarettes.

So generally accepted, medically, is this view of lung cancer and smoking that the present emphasis of preventive medicine has shifted from the obvious warnings regarding lung cancer to more subtle, but nonetheless important, areas where smoking has a deleterious effect.

In a joint statement published by the American Public Health Association, the American Heart Association, the American Cancer Society, and the National Tuberculosis Association, the following sentence appeared, "If it were possible to remove only one of the effects of cigarette smoke, the greatest contribution to health might be in eliminating the coronary heart disease hazard." They point out that this would cut the excess deaths due to smoking by about 50%. In terms of absolute values, deaths per 100,000 smokers are highest for coronary heart diseases, fewer for lung cancer, and even less for emphysema. This is mainly because coronary heart disease is much more common than the other two. It must be recalled, however, that smoking in relation to coronary heart disease is only one of the three or four chief contributing factors, while in relation to lung cancer and emphysema it is far and away the only significant factor.

Another area where smoking has an effect is on pregnant women and their offspring. In a British survey it was found that smokers have babies weighing about half a pound less than those born of non-smoking mothers. This is an important factor, for the trend medically is to define prematurity (which is a bad thing) by birth weight rather than by chronology. Additional effects such as increased frequency of stillbirths were also noted. Interestingly enough, in all these pregnant women, smoking as a factor itself seemed to have more effect than the number of cigarettes smoked.

In addition to other complications, it has been found that the heavy smoker has to work harder for the air he breathes. It seems that some minute particles in the smoke cause constriction of the air passages, which in turn leads to increased resistance to the passage of air, which finally leads to an increase in the work done by the lungs.

There are remote, unsuspected consequences of cigarette smoking also. While cigarette smoking probably doesn't cause stomach ulcers, it certainly makes the ulcer patient more symptomatic. One of New York City's leading abdominal surgeons won't operate personally on the ulcer of a patient who still smokes cigarettes because he feels the chances of recurrence of ulcer are very high in the cigarette smoker and he doesn't want to spoil the statistics of his operative cure rates!

There are other rarer conditions associated with cigarette smoking such as cancer of the larynx (voice box), cancer of the esophagus (gullet), cancer of the mouth and allied structures, and cancer of the urinary bladder, but these are all relatively rare.

What can be done about it? *Stop* smoking. "But, Doctor, that's very difficult." No one is denying that it's very difficult but it's not impossible. Consider this very telling fact: Most people, when they become ill with pulmonary disease, will either stop smoking or considerably reduce their consumption. This would indicate that, in general, people are aware of the relationship between cigarette smoking and disease and also that given the right motivation (which unfortunately, usually turns out to be fear), most people *can* "kick the habit" if they really want to.

As indication that they believe and practice what they preach, doctors (who see patients die every day of the consequences of heavy smoking) have, in the past 5 years, significantly diminished their cigarette consumption. Over 25% of doctors who smoked 5 years ago no longer smoke now.

Finally, let me quote again from the report I mentioned above, "Cigarette smoking is, without question, the greatest single public health problem this nation has ever faced ... Many of the diseases aggravated by cigarette smoking can be alleviated and those caused by smoking can be prevented. All members of the health community should collectively and individually accept the responsibility for doing their part in the prevention of diseases caused by personalized air pollution."

TONSILLECTOMIES

It wasn't too many years ago when it was nearly impossible for a red-blooded American boy or girl to reach his teens without having his tonsils removed. It was a sort of automatic rite of passage through childhood. It was "the thing" to do. It was almost to the point where not having your tonsils removed either meant that your parents were too poor to afford the operation or didn't know any better.

Obviously, this situation has changed drastically. Nowadays, only 20 to 30% of children have T&As (tonsillectomies and adenoidectomies—for in most cases when the tonsils are removed, the adenoids are removed at the same time). This still means 1 or 2 million T&As a year, and there actually is a significant body of physicians who believe that even that many T&As are too many and that probably only 2 to 10% of American children really need such an operation. And then there are the pediatricians in teaching hospitals and medical schools who feel that such surgery should rarely, if ever, be performed.

Some of the background of the value of tonsils and adenoids, if any, will help explain such a radical shift in medical opinion. I once heard a wise old doctor say, when the initial reports began to appear in the medical literature of the importance of such previously-assumed, "useless" organs such as the tonsils and the appendix, "It almost seems as if Whoever put the human body together may very well have known what He was doing." And the more we find out about the body, the more he is proving to be correct.

The tonsils are an important part of the lymph system which, in turn, is one of the most important systems of the body. As we evolved over the past couple of million years, we had to carry along in our bodies strong protection against foreign invasion—especially foreign living matter such as bacteria or viruses for if some other living organism were able successfully to implant itself in our bodies and began to grow there, the competition between it and us could prove to be so great that we might lose out. As a matter of fact, when a person dies of pneumonia or tuberculosis or other infectious disease, that is exactly what has happened. Some bug landed in us and got the upper hand: It thrives and we die.

For all of recorded and certainly prerecorded history, such has not, luckily, been the case for the majority of us. Sure, as we age and our "resistance" decreases, we contract and succumb to serious infections. But this always happens to less than 50% of us at any one time or we would not have survived as a species. For our protection against infections, therefore, the body has evolved two lines of defense: One is the humoral line and the other is the cellular line.

Briefly, the humoral line of defense consists of the multitude of substances that constantly float around in our blood—often the chief class of these substances is called antibodies—which prevent an invading foreign, infectious agent from gaining a foothold. The way they work seems to be a form of "memory-system": Once you've been significantly exposed to a certain virus, for example, the body makes a circulating memory chemical—the antibody—which specifically is shaped to control and kill the invader; and this memory-chemical often stays in our blood for the rest of our lives, ready to protect us against any future invasion by the organism that gave birth to this specific antibody.

The cellular line of the body defenses depends on two chief components: The lymph cells that circulate in the blood (these are cells that can be seen under the microscope in contrast to the nonvisible chemical substances which form the humoral line of defense) and the lymph nodes which are clusters of fixed lymph cells and lymph-cell forming tissue located in various portions of the body such as in the armpits, groin, neck area, *and* in the tonsils and appendix. These lymph cells either actively circulate to destroy foreign invaders or, in the case of the tonsils for example, destroy any such invader that might land there and try to multiply. This is especially important in the case of the tonsils for they stand guard on either side of the throat, the main portal of entry to the body—for all the air we breathe as well as all the food and drink we take in must pass the filter of the tonsils.

If the tonsils are so important, why was anyone taking them out in the first place? For one thing, it wasn't until relatively recently that their important defensive function was realized. For another, there were some children who had such frequent, severe, and recurrent throat infections that their tonsils became chronically enlarged. Not only did they enlarge, but they sometimes reached such massive proportions that they actually interfered with swallowing. And it was not at all uncommon that enlarged adenoids (which are lymph tissues up behind the soft palate, at the back of the nostrils) reached the point where they interfered with the ease of normal breathing through one's nostrils—so that these children became mouth breathers for the sake of comfort. Their faces could actually become permanently distorted from these blocking adenoids. Sometimes, removal of adenoids was recommended in the case of children who had frequent serious ear infections. Often, removal of the tonsils was advocated for children who had frequent, severe strep throat or throat abscesses—on the theory that removal helps diminish such episodes. Knowing as we do now the important function of the tonsils in combating infection, it is hard to understand how tonsillar removal could have *diminished* the frequency of infection.

What probably dealt the death blow to tonsillectomy frequency was not our recent understanding of the importance of their function; rather, two very interesting and somewhat disconcerting observations have been made and it seems (at least, so far) confirmed: Patients who had their tonsils removed had a greater chance of developing bulbar polio (which is the dreaded massively paralytic, often fatal, form of the disease) rather than the milder form of polio that developed in those who still have their tonsils. Of course, the removal of the tonsils does not *make* one get polio; rather, if you got.it, tonsillar absence was often associated with a severe form of the disease.

The other disquieting observation is that people who have their tonsils out have a three times greater likelihood of developing Hodgkin's disease in later life. Hodgkin's disease is a form of cancer of the lymph tissue that some doctors believe may have a virus either as its underlying cause or as a very important contributing factor. Therefore, one may reason that anything that protects us against virus infections in general "can't be all bad."

This is not to say that no one should have his tonsils removed. Most doctors choose, nowadays, a middle path: They wait until the child with chronic tonsillar problems is at least 5 years of age or older before recommending surgery. Often the enlarged tonsils will shrink after that age. Some doctors will wait even longer if breathing is in no way interfered with.

VARICOSE VEINS

One of the consequences of the evolutionary assumption of the upright posture by mankind has been an unusual, "unphysiologic," placing of a gravity pressure-stress upon veins in our lower extremities. In some people the consequence is that well-known complaint, varicose viens.

While all mankind walks upright, it is far from true that all mankind is subject to varicose veins. In many people, there is a strong family history of the condition; in other cases, the usual type of activity they do during the day may contribute to the condition: Thus, people who do a lot of prolonged standing—dentists, barbers, sales people in stores, etc.—are often more prone to the condition than those in more sedentary occupations. Tall people, probably because their height conveys a greater gravity pressure upon their lower extremities, are also more often subject to varicose veins than others. During the later stages of pregnancy, the abdominal pressure upon those veins is also considerably increased; and sometimes a permanent varicose vein condition can result.

The arteries are muscular tubes that carry blood away from the heart toward the most distal parts of the body; in effect, gravity cooperates with the arterial flow of blood. The veins, on the other hand, are thin, nonmuscular, quite "weak," blood vessels which serve to carry the blood back to the heart, and generally have to work against gravity to accomplish their task. If they are not able to use their own muscular contraction to get the blood back to the heart, how do they manage to do this? In the case of the big veins, they are usually buried deep among muscles; and the muscular contraction of the normal movements of the legs generally is adequate to help "milk" or squeeze the blood up the veins on its way back to the heart. A second line of defense against a gravity backup of blood in these thin-walled veins is the presence of one-way valves spaced at regular intervals along the course of these vessels. These valves allow the easy flow of blood back toward the heart, but they balloon out and snap together, effectively closing off the opening in the veins, if the blood tries to rush downward again.

What is commonly meant by varicose veins is a condition of dilated, tortuous, knotty, visible (and sometimes unsightly) veins of the legs. These veins are the superficial leg veins. The deep set of veins too can become varicose and cause symptoms but, being deep, is usually not visible because the vein valves are so situated that they prevent blood from the deep system from flowing back to the superficial veins.

The chief causes of varicose veins are: (1) the effects of postural strain, in persons whose vein valves are constitutionally defective and (2) any condition that causes obstruction of either the deep or the superficial venous blood flow so that enlargement of the superficial veins and formation of secondary channels occur. An example of the first cause would be in such an occupation as dentistry where the person has to stand most of the time and in one spot, so that he can't take too much advantage of the blood pumping action that his leg muscles would give if he were able to move around often and freely. Obviously, not all dentists have varicose veins for it takes a combination of the postural strain plus the inborn weakness or absence of the vein valves to cause them. As examples of the second cause of varicose veins, we have such internal body pressure-increasing conditions as pregnancy, abdominal tumors or fluid collections, and excessive weight.

The symptoms of varicose veins can vary all over the map. Probably the majority of people experiences no symptoms from them at all other than the fact that they're unhappy about the way their legs look. In others, especially after prolonged standing, there may be muscle cramps and increased fatigability of the leg muscles. Some may complain of an annoying sensation of tension and soreness at the back of the knee or over the areas of the varicose veins themselves. Sometimes ankle swelling can occur toward the end of the day, but this is usually gone after an overnight rest. Some women will only have symptoms around the time of their period (which is probably a manifestation of the pelvic congestion that occurs around that time).

More rarely, itching and eczemalike dermatitis called stasis dermatitis, either localized or generalized over the leg, may develop. Even pigmentation may appear over the involved areas of the leg, especially if there has been injury to the skin. Finally, but rarely, ulceration and even blood clots can occur.

When the only manifestation of varicose veins is the occurrence of those spiderlike, hair-thin, capillary bunches of discoloration with little if no localized swelling, no treatment is usually indicated. There is of course no harm in such persons using elastic stockings, but they are probably not needed. On the other hand, the use of elastic stockings or bandages is quite helpful for those who have the superficial, long, twisting, bulging veins with the symptoms of heaviness and tiredness but no signs of local skin breakdown present. When the complication of swelling of the lower leg begins, keeping the legs elevated by raising the feet at night so that the legs are higher than the heart is often recommended; and, if possible, such a maneuver should be performed intermittently during the day. Prolonged sitting and standing should be avoided since activity keeps those muscles exerting their "milking action" to help get the vein flow back toward the heart.

At one time, the injection of irritating chemicals was used for the treatment of varicose veins. They caused the offending veins to close off. Their use nowadays has given way in most cases to a surgical approach in the treatment of varicose veins. Here the veins are actually tied off, and as much of the offending parts as possible are stripped out and removed.

While such surgery is almost always going to be necessary in those persons who actually have skin breakdown as a consequence of their varicose veins, often a period of bed rest and soaks locally with or without the use of antibiotics are recommended in an attempt to achieve skin healing prior to the vein stripping.

UNNECESSARY ORGANS?

As modern research progresses, medical practice often finds itself in the uncomfortable position of having, figuratively, to eat its own words. Part of the body which had been assumed to be of no real use and were merely serving as modern remnants of our distant evolutionary past are turning out to have important functions—now, as well as then.

In the 1930's, the situation was such that if you were a self respecting parent and not absolutely "dirt-poor," you arranged for the automatic removal of your children's tonsils between the ages of 5–10. This accomplished a number of things: Most important of all it helped to keep up with the Joneses; it served to supplement the doctor's income; but unfortunately, it also served to traumatize the young victim both physically and psychologically. But, "the tonsils are of no use anyhow." Or so it was believed. Now, however, we know better. Tonsils are of very definite use, serving as one of the most important lines of defense of the body's protective mechanisms against invading organisms. Not only do the tonsils help protect the respiratory system from infections, but they even have remote protective effects that we are only beginning to learn about. Thus, in the days when polio was still a dreadful and prevalent disease, people whose tonsils had been removed prior to their contracting polio had a much higher chance of developing the dreaded, paralytic bulbar polio than those whose tonsils were still intact.

The appendix is also turning out to be an organ more sinned against than sinning. Long assumed to be of no use to the body, it was often routinely removed during the course of other operations. Very often, the doctor threw in its removal for free when operating as if he were doing you a favor, and again it was because medicine didn't know any better. The appendix, like the tonsils, is a very important part of the lymphatic defense system of the body; and its lymph cells are active in protecting us from outside invaders whether such invaders are infectious or otherwise. For example, a startling fact was revealed a few years ago when it was found that the incidence of cancer of the large intestine (that part of the intestine which is downstream from the appendix) was considerably higher in people who had previously had their appendices removed.

This is not to say that tonsils or appendices should never be removed; rather, they should not routinely be removed. Chronically infected, enlarged tonsils which are interfering with the child's breathing are a definite candidate for removal consideration. Only a madman would not remove an appendix afflicted by acute appendicitis.

The spleen, while not an organ which is removed routinely by anybody, is one about which comparatively little is known and little has only recently been discovered. We know that it serves as a mechanical graveyard for many of the aging cells of the circulation, but that did not seem to be a critical function. Now we are learning, however, that as part of the body's general lymphatic protective system, it has a very important function indeed, revealed only in its absence. Thus, the incidence of certain types of pneumonia, often rapidly fatal types to boot, is much higher in people whose spleens have had to be removed because of accidents, etc., than in those whose spleens are intact.

One organ that still remains on the rapidly dwindling list of useless organs is the gallbladder. We know that its chief function is to concentrate and store the bile fluids normally secreted by the liver. Nonetheless, its removal does not seen to interfere with liver function or digestion or any other function—for now. Who knows what tomorrow's medicine will reveal?

Finally, we come to the most mysterious organ in all of medicine: the pineal gland of the brain. For centuries although everybody seemed to know it was there, no one knew what it did. In certain types of newts and salamanders, it serves as a third eye on the top of their heads. One does hear occasionally of people who can see from the back of their heads, but one never hears of one who can see through the top of his head. Descartes, the French philosopher, believed that the pineal gland was the seat of the soul. While he has not been proved wrong, not too many people would go along with him nowadays. On the other hand, not too many people knew what the thing was doing in the brain in the first place. The very latest research has indicated that it may be a gland after all, and a very important one indeed, that may be involved with the endocrinology of sexual maturation. It may serve the critical function of secreting hormones which trigger other parts of the brain to secrete their hormones in turn.

HOW TO CHOOSE A DOCTOR

Perhaps one of the questions most frequently asked is how a person goes about obtaining the long- or short-term services of a physician: long-term in the sense of getting a family doctor, short-term for obtaining a specialist for a specific problem that may have arisen recently.

Even though the strides in medical knowledge over the past few decades have been tremendous, nonetheless, the problem of finding a personal physician may be even greater now in the age of super-specialization than it was in the "old days." However, the pattern of illness has not changed specifically among our population over these years: that is, a good 90% of visits to a physician do not require the administration of antibiotics, cortisone compounds, digitalis, insulin, or any other of the new and more powerful medications in the medical armamentarium.

Most visits to a physician stem from a concern about a problem which requires more of the doctor's expertise in ruling out serious conditions than in his having to apply some of the newer diagnostic or therapeutic techniques developed over the past few decades. However, there remain that 10% of people who do have serious medical problems and who need the very best and newest in diagnostic and therapeutic approaches. This latter group would have fared very poorly years ago before we had the new medications, and it is to them that the greatest rewards of medical progress can be offered.

With that as a background, how does one choose a doctor? A doctor is someone whom we should be able to turn to whenever we are afraid or worried about our health. Objectively, we may know that it is probably not serious, but at three o'clock in the morning, what if that hangnail is an early cancer? Our physician should be someone to whom we can respond as a person. Some patients are put off by the demonstrative, jolly, Dutch uncle approach, while others respond only to that. When choosing a family physician, one should not be ashamed to "shop around." We shop around for things like clothes and cars and houses; certainly we should not be loathe to shop around for the best health care for ourselves and our families.

One of the ideal qualities in a family physician is availability, and here we run into one of the chief complaints of modern day. "The answering service said he won't be in today." "This is his weekend off." "My doctor doesn't make house calls." There is no denying that the concept of the traditional, white-haired family doctor in his horse and buggy, who delivered the baby, took out the tonsils, was present at the young person's wedding, and then went on and delivered her baby, is probably a thing of the past. Let's not blame the medical community for this. What I have described briefly is an idealization of an image that was only too true in small town America 50 to 75 years ago. However, America is no longer "small town." Even our small towns are no longer "small town." The family doctor who made house calls and was almost a part of the family may have gone the way of the quilting bee. Personally, I'm not so sure that the passing of this kindly old man who used to make house calls is a good thing. So long as he was intelligently up-to-date with modern medical thinking, such a medical practitioner could offer outstanding service to that 90% we spoke of who didn't need digitalis, antibiotics, etc. Because, let's face it, even if you go to a superspecialist, while you may not come out with a superduper new remedy or test, you hopefully will come out with reassurance and peace-of-mind; and the old-time family doctor could give that probably better than anyone.

If, in your search for a good family physician, you should find that rare person who does make house calls or is otherwise often available to you and your family, cherish him—but wisely. The kindly old family doctor who makes house calls but doesn't know when to call in a specialist may be more of a menace than a help, but remember the need for the newest techniques of specialization occur in only about 10% of the people.

One good way to choose a family doctor after you have settled into an area is to find out whom the neighbors you like and trust use as their physicians. Often the local county Medical Society will be happy to supply you with the names of three physicians located close to your home.

For better or for worse, the general practitioner is steadily declining in American medicine, and the internist is taking his role as family physician. So, because the internist is a specialist, you may find that you will be using a specialist after all as your family doctor. Internal medicine, however, is a vast field with many sub-specialities, and the good family physician specialist should never be above calling in other specialists whenever the need arises. That, in a way, is one of the signs of a good doctor: He is not above calling in another specialist for another opinion or advice and certainly doesn't take it as a personal affront if you, the patient, make such a request. Many a doctor is pleased to comply with such a request because, in the long run, it may help solve the patient's problem; and a healthy, satisfied patient will usually be returning to such a physician.

If the need arises for a specialist, the best way to get one is to take the advice of the family physician you know and trust. He probably knows the local medical community better and more intimately than your friends and neighbors. For recommendations for a specialist, I would suggest that you rely on professional opinions. Again, let me emphasize that it's your health and your money. Therefore, don't be timid about changing specialists. There are so many people in each of the specialties and if, for whatever reason, the one recommended to you doesn't seem to be the right one for you, change. Ask your doctor for another specialist.

Finally, what about those individuals who are "never sick" and don't really need a doctor, so why have a family doctor? Because there is always the possibility that we might, on a Saturday afternoon, break a leg, or develop pneumonia, or have a heart attack, and it's either rely on the man with whom one has established contact or else go to a hospital Emergency Room, because it is almost impossible to obtain a doctor for the first time during the more traditional times when a doctor is not available, such as a Saturday afternoon. Let me hasten to add that going to a hospital Emergency Room is no longer the hit-and-miss type of medical care that it used to be some years ago. The majority of our hospitals nowadays have a full-time Emergency Room staff of very competent physicians who can take care of essentially all problems presented to them. So effective has this outlet become that many people use the hospital Emergency Room as their family doctor. While I don't think this is bad, I do think it is second best to establishing personal contact with a physician.

SUMMER ADVICE

Though no one really wants to get a bad sunburn, and everyone seems to know that one should get a gradual exposure to the sun, nonetheless many of us wind up with a really bad sunburn at the beginning of the season after all. It may be fine to know you are supposed to get 15 minutes of sun the first day, and then 30 minutes the second day, and 45 minutes to an hour the third day, but if you have a 1-week vacation coming up at the shore, you are not going to be too enthusiastic about following that regimen, which would entail spending most of your time indoors during the first half of your vacation week. Luckily, there now are some very effective sun screen lotions on the market which should be used by all of those who want to avoid severe burns and should especially be considered for the early exposures to the sun. Rather than recommend any specific trade names, let me suggest that you do a little label reading on your own to assure that you get a medically effective suntan lotion. Anything which has listed as one of its major ingredients para-aminobenzoic acid or, as some labels might carry it, PABA, while not giving you total 100% protection, should prove to be a most effective sun screen.

A mystique has grown up in America about the absolute necessity of salt tablets if one perspires, to the point where the ingestion of salt has become more of a ritual than a necessity. This usually will cause no problems except in persons with a tendency towards any kind of cardiovascular disease or high blood pressure, in which case any excess salt is of questionable value and may even be dangerous. For the normal person, though, there is no harm in the taking of salt even if it is taken unnecessarily. However, at the times when one is perspiring very heavily, it would not be a bad idea to take a little extra salt, either by sprinkling some on the food or in such items as saltine crackers. Many a salt tablet taker doesn't really know what he is taking it for—merely that it would probably prevent some dreadful condition. The reason one takes salt is that if you lose large quantities of salt through your sweat, the blood can become relatively salt depleted, leading to exhaustion, weakness, lightheadedness, a fall in blood pressure, and, even, in some cases, fainting. None of these are very frightening problems but they can be annoying, and so—salt.

An interesting fact for sunglass wearers is that if you really expect them to serve their purpose, which would be to filter out both ultraviolet and infrared rays, then they have to be made out of glass. Plastic lenses don't filter out infrared rays. The color of a sunglass is also important in filtering out light rays. Most tinted lenses are totally ineffective in providing glare protection except for those lenses which are neutral gray or sage green. Usually, a good sunglass is a prescription item, made specifically for you, and is not inexpensive. For those who don't need prescriptions, a glass lens with the requisite gray or green tint is ideal.

Some persons, luckily a minority, have relatively severe reactions to insect bits and stings. It is imperative that those persons take extra precaution to avoid exposure to recurrence of such bites. Certainly, no one goes around looking to be bitten; but these people should avoid those areas where the insect, to whose sting they are allergic, can be found. When most people are bitten or stung by an insect, they will get a little bit of redness and a lot of pain. That is a normal reaction. The people we are talking about here, however, are those who get a lot of redness, swelling, and puffiness of a large surrounding area after such exposure. These are the people who could get a severe respiratory reaction from a sting and, though it is rare, deaths have been reported from these accelerated allergic responses. It is probably true that once a person has had an accelerated allergic reaction to a bite or a sting, he is liable to experience another reaction of a similar or greater strength on future exposures.

Poison ivy sufferers are usually quite aware of the condition and know very well what to do to avoid future exposure. Nonetheless, for those who are exposed, in any case, vigorous washing of the involved part and clothing usually will help keep the condition under fairly good control. In a minority of people in whom the condition is very extensive and seems not to be getting under control even after 3 or 4 days, the current medical thinking is that small doses of cortisone compounds, usually by mouth, can be very effective if given for 4 or 5 days. The use of an antihistamine in poison ivy is still controversial. It may help and it certainly can do no harm.

For the gardeners among us, we should try to carefully wash all thorn wounds from rose thorns and other prickly objects. Some of these thorns can harbor a fungus that can cause lingering low grade infections of, for example, fingernails and fingers.

Athlete's foot generally tends to flourish in warm weather because our feet perspire more in warm weather. For those who are afflicted, sitting around with your shoes off, either in bare feet or just with your socks, in order to have that perspiration dry as much as possible is the ideal recommendation. There are various fungus medications that can be used to treat it, but it must be remembered that the basic cause is not the presence of the fungus but the presence of the moisture. If one's feet are not prone to much perspiration, just being exposed to the fungus will not cause athlete's foot. One way of keeping your feet dry is the frequent application of a nonirritating powder. Talcum powder is a good choice, and plain old baking soda may even be a better one since it has a reputation for absorbing odors besides being a drying agent.

Food poisoning is much more common in warm weather than in other times of the year since the bacteria multiply very rapidly as the temperature goes up. Picnics are also more common in warm weather than at any other time of the year, and so one should be careful to refrigerate adequately all foods that are going to be prepared but not served immediately, to keep them as cold as possible for as long as possible. While it is never a good idea to leave meats out on the stove to cool before refrigerating (refrigerators don't break down because a hot item is put into them), it is especially important that this practice be avoided in the summer months.

There still is some controversey as to the wisdom of going swimming after eating. It is known that in order to effectively absorb the products of digestion, we need a greatly increased volume of blood going to the gastrointestinal area for at least an hour or so after a meal. If one is swimming, one needs a lot of blood going to one's extremities; and it is quite possible that one's body would shunt its blood away from the stomach area, thus interfering to varying degrees with digestion. It is not at all clear, however, that the reverse is true, that the stomach would actually draw so much blood away from the extremities that one would get cramping in the extremities because digestion is overcoming their blood needs. So, if only not to interfere with normal digestive processes, it may still be a good idea to wait an hour or so after significant food intake before going into the water.

TRAVELER'S TIPS

It used to be that the primary requirement for a would-be traveler was to make sure that his smallpox vaccination certificate was up-to-date. However, thanks to the World Health Organization's massive attack on smallpox, the disease has been virtually eliminated. But if you're traveling to Ethiopia or nearby Somalia (the last places in the world where smallpox has been reported and where there may still be a few cases), you might want to check with your local board of health to see if you would require a smallpox vaccination after all. Do not rely on a blanket recommendation for vaccination on the part of your travel agent. Some of their recommendations are very out of date. In general, however, almost no one needs a smallpox vaccination anymore.

Other immunizations about which your board of health can bring you up to date are for cholera, yellow fever, and polio when necessary.

Once again, these apply only to very limited areas of the globe. Up-to-date information is necessary since last year's infected area may be this year's disease-free area.

The question often comes up as to whether or not one should receive gamma globulin shots to help ward off infectious hepatitis. The current public health recommendations are that unless one is going to be staying for a prolonged time (usually 3 months) in a certain area, the gamma globulin shots are not necessary.

Many people have their own set of favorite medicines which they take fairly regularly. Naturally these should be taken along. The question comes up, however, about various types of prophylactic medicines for travel. Aspirin is not a bad idea. It is also wise to take along a good antidiarrheal medication (the better ones require a doctor's prescription). For those who have a tendency to become airsick or seasick, a medicine to help control that is advisable. Should one take along antibiotics? My own feeling is no. For one thing, diseases which require antibiotics are the exception rather than the rule. For another, if a person gets sick enough that antibiotics should be considered (for example, controlling high fever, a kidney infection, a serious respiratory infection, or in unremitting diarrhea), it is better to consult a local physician for diagnosis and treatment than just to take blindly some nonspecific antibiotic one may have carried along from home. Very often the local physician will have seen similar cases and will be fully equipped to handle your special problem.

Perhaps the most frequent of all the problems encountered by travelers is diarrhea. If ever the old adage was true, surely it is in the case of diarrhea that an ounce of prevention is worth a pound of cure. If you take (especially in exotic places or developing nations) some reasonable precautions in drinking and eating, you may get away home free.

All tap water, both hot and cold, should be treated as suspect. Don't even use it to brush your teeth and above all, don't accept it in ice cube form. The mere presence of alcohol (if the ice cubes are to be used in drinks) does not guarantee the killing of infectious organisms in contaminated ice cubes. So, what do you drink? If the water has been boiled, hot coffee and tea are fine. Beer and wine are usually all right. Some authorities feel that soft drinks should be avoided; others feel that they are safe, especially if the country is a little more developed. Milk is a big question mark. Some places do not pasteurize; and even in those places which do, improper bottling and capping may lead to problems. When it comes to water itself, boiled water is fine if you have personally boiled it. If you can't boil it, various methods of purification are available. Halazone tablets or Globaline tablets can be used. Some authorities suggest traveling with a small bottle of bleach and an eye dropper. One drop of bleach per quart of water or two drops if the water is cloudy will usually kill most bacteria within 10 minutes. Others suggest two or three drops of iodine per quart of water to achieve the same effects. Sometimes, to be absolutely safe, the water should be filtered first and then boiled.

What do you eat? Generally, you're always safe with cooked, hot foods (here, hot is not used in the sense of "spicy"). Fish, meat, and vegetables should all be served hot, and meat should be preferably well done, regardless of how you might like it at home. All raw food, especially vegetables, should be avoided. The only fruits or vegetables that should be eaten are those you can peel yourself. Beware of fancy, lavish buffets served on terraces or patios. (They may have been out a long time or refrigerated on a bed of contaminated ice.) Cold plates should be avoided as well as custards, cream pastries, and potato salads. One authority has recommended that one not accept smoking, salting, pickling, or drying of meat as a substitute for thorough cooking.

If you need a physician while abroad, the travel agent or the American Embassy or Consulate can usually provide you with the names of qualified physicians or hospitals.

Finally, what about jet lag? Although a popular diagnosis a few years ago, one hears less about it nowadays. Nonetheless, here are some tips. For short flights, eat, go to bed, and arise the first day or so according to home time. When traveling west to east, go to bed progressively earlier before the trip; and vice versa east to west. Use food and drink sparingly during the flight and the first 3 days after travel. Arrange your schedule to shorten the day rather than the night.

Regardless of where you have been, you should see a doctor if you develop a fever or diarrhea after returning home.

DRIVING ACCIDENTS

A letter in a recent medical journal suggested that the primary cause of a large percentage of otherwise unexplained driving accidents is narcolepsy, which is an abnormal tendency to fall asleep during inactivity or during monotonous activity. The sleep may last from moments to minutes and like ordinary sleep (and, therefore, unlike unconsciousness) can be terminated immediately by appropriate stimulation. It can also be prevented by simple measures such as change of posture or conversation. The danger is that sufferers from this condition can fall asleep without realizing it.

The exact frequency of narcolepsy as a medical factor in causing driving accidents may not be settled yet, but this recent medical journal note may very well serve as a stimulus to review some known medical factors in driving accidents.

California is one of 17 states that regulates the driving privileges of persons with specific chronic medical conditions. A recent survey of such registered persons in California revealed that drivers with medical conditions had significantly higher accident and violation rates at all ages (up to twice as many accidents per million miles of driving) than did those in the comparison sample of "normals." These chronic medical conditions included not only epilepsy and alcoholism, which one would have expected, but also high blood pressure and other cardiovascular diseases, diabetes, Parkinsonism, severe arthritis, and various forms of psychotic mental illnesses, which are generally unexpectedly implicated medical factors.

Of course, health defects should be kept in proper perspective in relation to traffic accidents. In most accidents in which the driver is at fault, it is not because he is ill or alcoholic. The fault lies with the healthy person who is careless or reckless and with the moderate drinker who fails to recognize the effects of alcohol on his alertness, judgment, and speed of his reflexes. As a matter of fact, an interesting note was brought to light recently. Most persons in whom alcohol was a significant factor in their driving accidents were *not* alcoholics but rather were "normals" who had just had "a little too much to drink." The rationalization that "well, I can certainly have this drink; after all, I'm not an alcoholic" is a dangerous and false reassurance. Let's not forget that according to the National Safety Council, drinking is involved in *not less than 50% of fatal motor accidents.* It has been stated in a recent medical journal "that unidentified alcoholism is perhaps the most important single human variable correlated with serious to fatal accidents."

Some other factors found to be of significance in driving accidents include age under 30 or over 59. However, the presence of the medical conditions mentioned above in the latter group made them even more significantly liable to have driving accidents. Sex was also found to be a factor since, in 1964, females were involved in only 78% of the number of male driving accidents. Also important is the fact that those with a past history of accident or violation are more likely to have another episode than those without such a history.

Attempts at preventing highway accidents are being properly focused on improvements in automotive design and equipment and on highway engineering. Attention is also being paid to driver training and to the psychological factors that may impair a driver's performance. It is now evident that a broad view of the various medical conditions mentioned above that may affect the physical fitness of the driver is also required. Hopefully, the pointing out of the significance of such conditions will lead to an awareness that will manifest itself as extra caution, in addition to careful medical management to check the disorder.

Getting back, in closing, to narcolepsy, one medical journal recently suggested adding two slogans to "don't drive after drinking": "Don't drive if you feel sleepy" and "if you tend to fall asleep unexpectedly, see your doctor."

Index

hypertension, 22
donors, 114–115
failure, 113
infection, 106
  back problems, 232
  sickle-cell anemia, 4
  underweight, 192
polycystic, 113
stones, and back problems, 232

Laryngeal cancer, and smoking, 278
Laryngitis, 154
Laryngoscopy, 265
Laxatives, 94–95
Leptospirosis, 146
Leukemia, 11
  lymph node enlargement, 271
  statistics, 13
  use of platelets, 3
  use of white blood cells, 3
  viral cause, 12
Librium, 219
Liver
  biopsy, 93
  cancer, 12
  disease
    amebiasis, 167
    anemia, 9
    hemorrhoids, 44
  use of albumin, 2
Liver fluke infestations, 169
Lockjaw. See Tetanus
LSD, 212–214
Lumbago, 232
Lung
  cancer, 11–14, 18
    and smoking, 276
  function of, 241–242
Lung fluke infestations, 168
Lupus erythematosus, as autoimmune
  disorder, 190
Lymph nodes, 269–272
Lymphoma, 11
  and lymph node enlargement, 271
Lymph system
  appendix, 89
  resistance to diseases, 280
  tonsils, 279

Malignant melanoma, 11, 63

Malnutrition, use of albumin, 2
Mammography, 16
Marijuana, 212–214
Massage, in bursitis, 240
Mastectomy, 17
Mastoid infections, and dizziness, 205
Maturity–onset diabetes, 171
Measles
  gamma globulin, 2
  immunization, 136, 138
Medications, and lymph node enlargement,
  271
Meniere's disease, 205
Meningitis, 209
Menopause, and cystic mastitis, 256
Methyl alcohol. See Wood alcohol
Migraine, 206, 214–215
Miltown, 219
Miner's elbow, 239
Moles, 61–63
Mononucleosis, infectious (glandular fever),
  142–145
  and lymph node enlargement, 271–272
Morphine, 219
Mortality statistics, 37
Multiple sclerosis, 215–218
  and dizziness, 205
Mumps
  gamma globulin, 2
  immunizations, 136, 138
  sterility, 136
Myocardial infarction. See Coronary heart
  disease
Myopia. See Nearsightedness
Myxedema. See Hypothyroidism

Narcolepsy, 295
Narcotics, and driving, 77
Nasal allergy, 153
Nasal polyps, 149, 152
National Council on Alcoholism, 71
Nearsightedness (myopia), 84
Nerve disease, in diabetes, 170
Nerve pressure, and back problems, 234
Neuralgia, trigeminal, 210
Niacin deficiency (pellagra), 198
Night blindness, and vitamin A deficiency,
  194
Nun's knee, 239